The Zika Virus Handbook

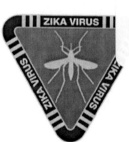

The Zika Virus Handbook

A DOCTOR EXPLAINS ALL YOU NEED TO KNOW ABOUT THE PANDEMIC

❖ ❖ ❖

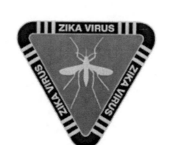

Joseph Alton, MD

1305828

DISCLAIMER

The information given and opinions voiced in this volume are for educational and entertainment purposes only and do not constitute medical advice or the practice of medicine. No provider-patient relationship, explicit or implied, exists between the publisher, author, and readers. This book does not substitute for such a relationship with a qualified provider. The author and publisher strongly urge their readers to seek modern and standard medical care with certified practitioners whenever and wherever it is available.

The reader should never delay seeking medical advice, disregard medical advice, or discontinue medical treatment because of information in this book or any resources cited in this book.

Although the authors have researched all sources to ensure accuracy and completeness, they assume no responsibility for errors, omissions, or other inconsistencies therein. Neither do the authors or publisher assume liability for any harm caused by the use or misuse of any methods, products, instructions, or information in this book, or any resources cited in this book.

All images via shutterstock.com
Copyright 2016 Doom and Bloom, LLC
Print ISBN-13: 9780988872585
E-book ISBN-10: 978-0-9888725-9-2
ISBN 10: 0988872587

This book is dedicated to mothers everywhere. Their commitment to the next generation is unyielding and timeless. It is the reason I feel blessed to have had the privilege of caring for pregnant women during my career as an obstetrician.

Joseph Alton, MD, FACOG

About Joseph Alton, MD

JOSEPH ALTON, MD IS A Life Fellow of the American College of Ob/ Gyn and Retired Fellow of the American College of Surgeons. After a 25 year career as an advocate for the health of pregnant women, he now devotes his time to speaking on the subject of epidemic and disaster medical preparedness.

His NY Times Bestseller in Health "The Ebola Survival Handbook" and his 3-category #1 Amazon bestselling book "The Survival Medicine Handbook" are considered informative guides to help inform those who wish to be prepared for the epidemics and disasters that too often dominate the news.

Dr. Alton is a member of the Wilderness Medical Society and has been featured in the NY Times, The Miami Herald, Tulsa World, Glenn Beck, Dana Loesch, Mother Jones, American Survival Guide, and various ABC, CBS, NBC, BBC, and Fox affiliates. He is a frequent contributor to several leading magazines writing about disaster preparedness and austere medicine. His website at www.doomandbloom.net has more than 800 articles, videos, and podcasts on medical preparedness.

Table of Contents

Introduction:
A Family's Heartbreak

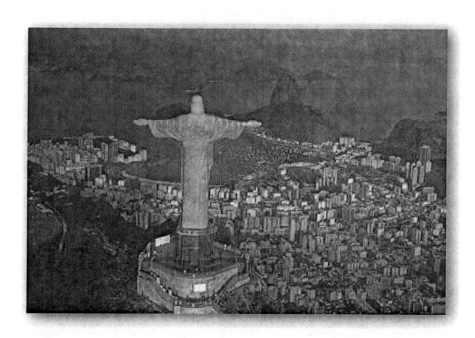

Lucia Barbosa of Recife, Brazil was just like any other young woman looking forward to having her first baby. She had married a young bricklayer and anticipated having a large family like the one she came from.

Lucia had to wait a while for her first appointment to a midwife in her area. Her first exam showed her to be about 18 weeks pregnant and she was excited to find that her due date came right around Christmas. Except for some morning sickness and a little back pain, she was feeling fine. She was given prenatal vitamins and an appointment was set up for her first ultrasound.

Lucia and her husband were excited to have a chance to "see" the baby. They arrived for the ultrasound appointment at 20 weeks along and were thrilled to see their baby move and were relieved to see that it had all its fingers and toes. It was even suggested to them that it looked like it might be a boy. His name would be Afonso, which means "noble king".

This is where the happy part ends. Part of the ultrasound exam involves measuring the various parts of the fetus. Everything was normal until the technician measured the head circumference of the baby. The first measurement seemed off, but three measurements are usually performed. All three seemed unusually small, and the technician kept measuring again and again, thinking that she might just have the wrong angle. Every way she checked, however, the answer was the same. The baby's head was too small.

Lucia and her husband were worried. Everyone wants a perfect baby; maybe the results were wrong. The midwife sent her to see an obstetrician, and then one of the few subspecialists in maternal-fetal medicine in the region. They assured her that they would follow the baby's growth and see how it develops.

Unfortunately, repeated ultrasounds kept showing a lag in the growth of the baby's head. The doctors reviewed her history, but she had been healthy, except for a mild "cold" she had experienced the month before her first appointment. She was achy and had a slight fever, but it went away after a few days and she thought little of it.

The doctors didn't believe it was a factor. After all, many women get colds when they're pregnant and have perfectly normal babies. This baby, however, was definitely not normal.

It finally came time to deliver the baby. The labor was uneventful, even easy, compared to many others. Lucia was thrilled to have the baby in her arms, but when she took a good look at it for the first time, it didn't seem normal. The head was, indeed, very small and the baby was whisked away by labor room staff for further evaluation.

It turned out that Afonso had a rare condition called "microcephaly". The baby developed seizures, and was transferred to a larger hospital. When the parents visited their baby, they were given the news that Afonso may have significant developmental disabilities, but would survive.

After a time, the baby stabilized and reached the point where it could go home. Lucia was told that her baby would require normal baby care for now, but that she could expect her son to need special help, perhaps for the rest of its life. Lucia cried.

Lucia Barbosa isn't a real person, but her story is very real for thousands of women. Ordinarily, the birth of a baby like Afonso would be a rare event in Brazil. Although a large and youthful country, only about 150 of the multitude of babies born each year have microcephaly. This year, however, things are different. Babies with the deformity are being born all over in much greater numbers. At present, the number is more than 4000 in Brazil alone.

Microcephaly is a condition that causes abnormalities in brain and cranial development which last a lifetime. A large number of cases of this birth defect can severely tax the resources of underdeveloped countries that must deal with the problem.

As a Life Fellow of the American College of OB/GYN, I delivered babies that were born with a number of abnormalities, including microcephaly. The human race isn't perfect, and we don't always produce perfect babies. Thankfully, most of my patients had normal infants, but one or two per cent of pregnant women have babies with congenital (birth-related) issues.

You can only imagine the emotional toll on a family with a baby born with microcephaly. The full extent of the disability in each case is often not known until the child fails to reach developmental milestones. Already, affected families in Brazil are feeling the stigma associated with a child that appears "deformed" and may have very limited potential.

What's causing this huge spike in abnormal newborns? Some were born with other deformities as well as microcephaly; a number did not survive. Tests were done post-mortem for every possible cause.

The researchers noted that many women had a "cold" during the pregnancy. Testing for various infectious diseases testing was performed after the fact to be sure that every possible cause was investigated.

The results came out that a little-known virus called Zika showed up in some of the tests. Zika virus (ZIKV) was an infection previously unknown in the Western Hemisphere, having originated in Africa, Asia, and Polynesia. Now, however, it's clear that it had crossed the Atlantic, apparently carried by mosquitoes. Cases are being reported throughout Central and South America, as well as the Caribbean.

Did Zika virus cause microcephaly in young Afonso and thousands of other newborns? If so, is it the next pandemic? The World Health Organization thinks so, describing it as "spreading explosively" and an "international public health emergency".

The WHO now suggests that there may be millions of Zika virus cases upcoming in the New World, and that 1.5 million may already have been infected (mostly without signs or symptoms).

Some cases of acute Zika disease will occur in those expecting a baby. The WHO predicts that over 100,000 newborns may be affected throughout the regions that ZIKV has been identified.

In Brazil alone, there are half a million women pregnant at any one point in time. Thousands of cases of acute ZIKV have been identified in pregnant women in Colombia, and more are suspected in Venezuela.

In the mostly Catholic countries of South America, abortion is often forbidden by law except in cases of rape or to save the life of the mother. This means that any abnormal baby is likely to be born and must be cared for by the state.

Given the serious nature of the consequences, even the Pope, leader of the world's Catholics, has loosened restrictions on practicing birth control in the epidemic zone (although not on termination of a pregnancy).

Acute Zika virus disease has already been identified in the United States from New York to Hawaii. Cases of microcephaly have been extremely rare, but the Aedes mosquito ranges over vast swaths of U.S. territory. In recent times, it has already been responsible for a number of cases of related viral infections in the U.S., such as Chikungunya and Dengue Fever.

This book is meant to educate the public about Zika virus, its history, presentation, and what can be done to prevent the illness and its effects. Related viral diseases will be discussed as well, and you will learn a great deal about pandemic disease in general.

The Zika question must be approached calmly, rationally, and without panic. A plan of action is necessary, however, if we are to prevent the heartbreaking consequences that many families must suffer, often for the rest of their children's lives.

PART 1

What is Zika Virus?

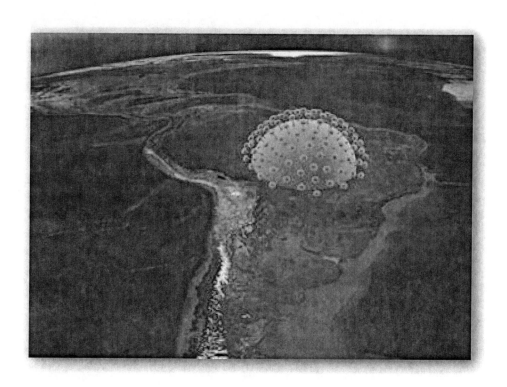

The History of Zika

IN TODAY'S WORLD OF HIGH technology, we have seen success in the treatment and prevention of many infectious diseases. Although we have had success curing many illnesses with antibiotics, we are still struggling with outbreaks caused by viruses. In 2014, thousands died in West Africa during the Ebola epidemic. In 2015, Chikungunya virus crossed the Atlantic into the Western Hemisphere and infected up to two million people.

Zika virus (ZIKV) has become the latest pandemic, and the first to generate travel warnings specifically for women that are pregnant or of childbearing age. Previously unknown to citizens of the Americas, The World Health Organization states that it may affect up to four million people and possibly be the cause of many babies born with lifelong disabilities.

What is Zika virus? Zika virus (ZIKV) is a member of the *Flavivirus* family, which contains a number of well-known diseases such as Yellow Fever, Chikungunya, Dengue Fever, and West Nile virus. Zika is named after the the Zika Forest of Uganda near Lake Victoria, where the virus was first identified in 1947 in a rhesus macaque monkey.

In the 1950s, the single-stranded RNA virus was first isolated in humans. Isolated cases were found at first, but since 2007, outbreaks have occurred in Africa, India, Southeast Asia, and the Polynesian Islands. Studies in these areas found that a widespread population carried antibodies against the virus, which suggests that it has existed, unidentified, for a much longer time.

There appear to be two strains of ZIKV, one from Africa and one from Asia. It has been hypothesized that the Asian version traveled with mosquitoes that followed international visitors to the 2014 World Cup in Rio de Janeiro, Brazil, and other cities. An outbreak in the Polynesian Islands in 2014 may have served as a way-station.

Due to its novelty, Zika Virus is spreading rapidly through the Western Hemisphere. The populations affected have had little chance to develop immunity. All age groups are vulnerable, even healthy young adults.

ZIKV isn't only thought by some researchers to have a relationship to birth defects like the unfortunate newborn in the introduction to this book. It is also associated with Guillain-Barre syndrome, a condition in which the body's immune system attacks its own nerve cells. These victims suffer muscle weakness and paralysis that might be temporary or permanent. In some case, it is fatal.

In the United States, the grand majority of Zika cases are seen in those who have recently returned from countries where there are ongoing outbreaks. As the mosquito that spreads the virus can live in certain regions of the U.S., ZIKV is expected to eventually show its presence in locally transmitted cases.

Future spread is also predicted as a result of the highly-anticipated 2016 Summer Olympic Games, which will be held in Brazil, the epicenter of the current epidemic. As well, Rio de Janeiro, Brazil is the site for the wildly popular Carnival event, held yearly.

Zika may have an impact that is more than medical. With many countries issuing warning to their citizens to avoid travel to places where there are ZIKV outbreaks, a negative effect on economies dependent on tourism is sure to occur. Similar warnings given during the Ebola epidemic of 2014 devastated the financial fortunes of many West African countries.

Even more devastating to a country's future might be the recommendation that nations like El Salvador are giving to female citizens: Don't get pregnant for the next two years. Jamaica has given the same warning for the next 12 months. Even the Philippines has recommended that women avoid becoming pregnant until more is known about Zika virus.

Now countries far from the current Zika virus epidemic are reporting cases, mostly from travelers to South America. Countries that couldn't be farther away from the outbreak zone, like Russia and China, are reporting active cases of the acute illness.

The United States is adding guidelines to include those who are sexual partners of women at risk, and also to limit the possibility that Zika virus might make its way to blood banks through donors who have recently visited the epidemic zone.

How Does Zika Virus Spread?

Zika virus is one of many infectious diseases transmitted from the bites of mosquitoes. A species that can pass a pathogen (disease-causing organism) to humans is called a "vector". Mosquitoes serve that purpose for many diseases, such as malaria. The Aedes family of mosquitoes, in particular, has been singled out as the most likely agent of spread of the Zika virus.

The equatorial countries where Zika was first found have some factors in common: warm weather, large areas of stagnant, standing water, large mosquito populations, and poor sanitation.

With commercial air travel so freely available, it makes sense that the Aedes mosquito could easily hitchhike its way to the New World. Once in the Western Hemisphere, many countries (such as Brazil) offer a welcoming environment for the mosquito to thrive. Some of these mosquitoes carried the Zika virus to a population with little immunity against it.

Despite this, it wasn't until May of 2015 that Zika cases started showing up in South America. Spread was rapid, and now the virus can be found in just about every country in the hemisphere. If an Aedes mosquito can live in a place, it can carry and transmit ZIKV there.

Although mosquito-borne transmission is, by far, the most common way to contract Zika virus, cases of transmission from human to human through sexual contact have been reported.

A researcher traveled to Senegal in Africa to study mosquitoes and suffered several bites. He returned to the United States and developed Zika symptoms, but not before having sexual relations with his wife. She subsequently developed the illness. This became the first proven case of an insect-borne virus passed though intercourse.

As a result of this case and a number of others, the United States has issued a warning and some specific recommendations for men traveling from Zika-affected areas. If a man has a pregnant partner he should either abstain from sex, or use condoms, until the end of his partner's pregnancy.

In addition, researchers suspect transmission through blood transfusions and found evidence that the virus may exist in saliva samples. Although ZIKV remains in the blood for only a week or so, it is unknown how long it may stay in semen or other bodily fluids. In the case of Ebola, male survivors were found to still have evidence of the virus in the semen several months after recovery.

The most serious human transmission is from mother to fetus, and this is the method that causes the most concern. Zika has been found in the amniotic fluid of a number of pregnancies, proving that the virus can pass through the placenta. It may also be possible to pass it to a newborn at the time of birth if the mother is ill. No reports of Zika passed through breastfeeding currently exist, however.

As we learn more about Zika virus, it may become clear that it can be spread in more ways than currently known. We are only in the beginning stages of research into the virus, its effects, and what can be done to treat and prevent it.

The Aedes Mosquito

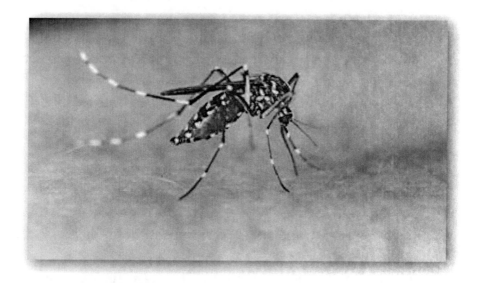

If you were asked, "What is the most dangerous animal on the planet?", you might think of the great white shark, the crocodile, or the tiger. You'd be wrong. It's the mosquito.

There are over 3500 species of mosquitoes on the planet, and many of them have a beneficial effect on the environment, such as pollinating certain plants and serving a food source for birds, fish, and other small animals. The United States has 176 species.

A number of species are truly dangerous, however, such as the Anopheles mosquito that transmits Malaria, a disease caused by a parasite called Plasmodia. Malaria causes millions of deaths every year in underdeveloped tropical countries.

In addition to Malaria, a number of serious viral diseases are passed to humans by mosquitoes. The mosquitoes that are most associated with viral disease are members of the Aedes family.

The name of the Aedes mosquito comes from the Greek word for "unpleasant". They originally made their home in tropical and sub-tropical zones. Now, however, they can be found everywhere in the world except for Antarctica. Most species can be identified by a pattern of white and black body markings.

Aedes Aegypti is the species most known to transmit the Zika virus in Africa and Asia. It is also considered the mosquito most likely to carry ZIKV in the New World. Unlike some other mosquitoes, it has a distinct preference for human hosts as opposed to animals.

It was first discovered in the 1700s, and has played a role in many epidemics. *Aedes Aegypti* passed Yellow Fever to workers during the construction of the Panama Canal, and was responsible for the Chikungunya pandemic that struck the Western Hemisphere in 2014-5.

Others in the same family, like the Asian Tiger mosquito (*Aedes Albopictus*), have recently crossed the Atlantic and can also spread Zika and other viral diseases. Asian Tiger mosquitoes are always on the search for a victim but, unlike other mosquitoes, are cautiously persistent when it comes to their blood meal. They often break it off short without enough blood ingested for the development of their eggs. You might think this is a good thing, but the result is that Asian tiger mosquitoes bite multiple hosts instead of just one. This makes them particularly efficient at transmitting diseases from person to person.

The fact that they bite different species enables the Asian tiger mosquito to be a vector for certain viruses and other disease causing organisms that can jump species boundaries. West Nile Virus is one example.

Most mosquitoes prefer to bite at dawn and dusk, but both *Aedes Aegypti* and *Aedes Albopictus* are aggressive biters all day long. They feed less often at night. These insects prefer shady areas to rest and may even live indoors, but can handle prolonged exposure to the sun if human hosts are available.

DIFFERENCES BETWEEN MALE AND FEMALE MOSQUITOES

Mosquitoes generally feed on sugars, but the female Aedes mosquito must have a blood meal to develop its eggs and reproduce. Therefore, only the female has any need to bite humans.

Besides the fact that only female mosquitoes bite humans, there are other visible differences between male and female Aedes mosquitoes:

* The male mosquito's mouth parts are somewhat smaller than the females.
* Like most insects, mosquitoes have antenna. The hairs on the mosquitoes' antenna allow them to hear. The male's antennae are "feathery" and larger than that of the female. This is because the male uses it to find females.
* Generally, male mosquitoes are smaller than females.
* Males live shorter lives than females.

WHAT ATTRACTS AEDES MOSQUITOES?

Mosquitoes are attracted by certain substances that are emitted by mammals. Carbon Dioxide is a powerful attractant when it is exhaled by humans, and mosquitoes can "smell" it up to 50 yards away. It's thought by some that pregnant women may exhale more carbon dioxide than others.

Movement and heat will also attract mosquitoes, as well as certain compounds on the skin, such as cholesterol, uric acid, and even lactic acid from sweat.

THE LIFE CYCLE OF THE AEDES MOSQUITO

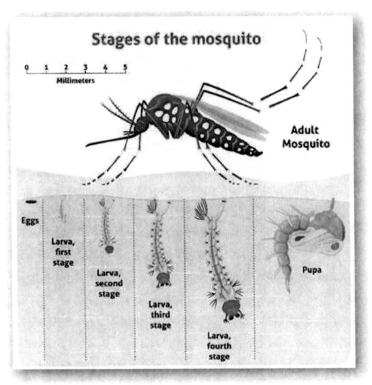

The life cycle of *Aedes aegypti*, like other mosquitoes, show dramatic changes in habitat and shape. Female lay their eggs on moist surfaces above the water line on plants, but may even utilize the inner walls of flower vases or discarded jars. They produce about 100 eggs at a time.

These eggs are very hardy. They remain stuck to the surface like glue and can survive up to a year, even if dry. This gets them through winters in temperate climates.

Once the eggs are covered with water from rainfall (or by humans), they hatch. The worm-like juveniles (known as "larvae") look nothing like the adult. They feed on microbes and organic matter.

Larvae must go through several stages called "instars", where they molt (shed their skins) as they grow. Although the larvae live in water, they need air to breathe. They come up to the surface from time to time to take in a supply through a siphon in the back of their bodies.

Once the larvae reach the fourth instar, they become a "pupa". During this stage, the body floats on the surface and breathes through tubes called "trumpets". Over one to four days, it changes into a fully formed adult mosquito. Once metamorphosis is complete, they emerge from the pupal skin as fully adult mosquitoes. A short period of rest is then necessary at the water's surface for the body to harden. The whole process from egg to adult happens in 8-10 days at warm temperatures.

After feeding from a human host, the young adult female Aedes mosquito will begin to look for water sources to lay eggs. During her lifetime of 2-4 weeks, she'll never go more than a few city blocks from her birthplace.

Despite this, the Aedes mosquito has found its way onto commercial aircraft and ocean-going freighters, carrying diseases like Zika, Yellow Fever, Dengue Fever, and Chikungunya. It's hardy, aggressive, and on the move.

Signs and Symptoms

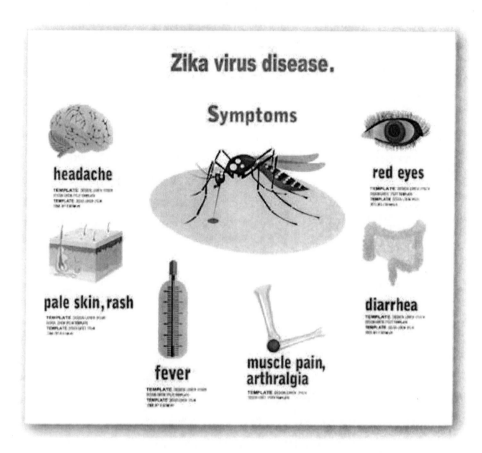

For a disease with heartbreaking consequences for newborns, Zika virus is a relatively mild illness when a person is first infected. After being bitten by a mosquito, there is a period of time where no symptoms appear. This is called the "incubation period". Although the exact incubation period of Zika is not known for certain, it is thought to be several days to a week or more.

The most common symptoms of Zika are fever, headaches, fatigue, and a patchy rash. The rash starts in the face and moves down the body. Many victims also experience joint or muscle pain and some even develop conjunctivitis (also known as "pink eye"). Occasionally, there have been reports of diarrhea or other bowel disturbances. Few of these symptoms require hospitalization and deaths are very rare. After a few days to a week, the patient recovers.

It should be noted that there are no symptoms whatsoever in the grand majority (80%) of those infected. Although this underscores the mild nature of the acute illness, the lack of signs could be ominous for the pregnant woman: She won't know that she had the infection until ultrasound results reveal abnormal fetal development.

GUILLAIN-BARRE SYNDROME

Despite the generally mild nature of ZIKV disease, a small percentage will develop a more serious condition known as Guillain-Barre syndrome. In Guillain-Barre, the body's immune system attacks the protective coverings of its own nerve cells (the "myelin sheaths"). The signs and symptoms occur a few days to weeks after the patient experiences a respiratory or gastrointestinal viral infection.

Guillain-Barré is called a "syndrome" rather than a specific disease because it may be caused by a number of different pathogens (disease-causing organisms). A syndrome is a condition characterized by a collection of signs and symptoms. As these may be variable from person to person, it is difficult to identify in its earliest stages. As the conditions slows down signals traveling along nerves, certain tests like Nerve Conduction Velocity (NCV) measurements can give health professionals results that might aid the diagnosis.

Guillain-Barre syndrome causes nerve damage that leads to muscle weakness in extremities and, occasionally, paralysis requiring life support.

Other symptoms include:

- Numbness and tingling in the hands, feet, and mouth
- Weakness in facial muscles
- Difficulty swallowing
- Slurred speech
- Pain, especially in the back muscles
- Shortness of breath (severe cases)
- Blood pressure issues and irregular heartbeats

Strange sensation in fingers and, more often, toes usually are the first symptoms, leading to extremity weakness that spreads from the legs to the arms and upper body over several days. These symptoms become so severe in some cases that certain muscles cannot be used at all. Paralysis may last for weeks. In the worst cases, difficulty breathing may require advanced support. Even the heart beat and blood pressure may be difficult to maintain. In some cases, the patient may die. Luckily, most sufferers will recover, but it is often a long and difficult process. Full recovery may take 3-6 months.

Diagnosis

Zika virus is difficult to diagnose, as the symptoms are mild and similar to many other minor infections. The potential for misdiagnosis is very high. Indeed, the acute illness is often gone by the time the average person can get in to see their doctor.

Even those who present to their physician while they are experiencing the acute illness are unlikely to be correctly diagnosed. Before, this was because of lack of information about this little-known virus. Now that Zika has caught the attention of the medical profession, the index of suspicion may be higher, but there are still major obstacles to making the correct diagnosis.

At present, there are no commercially-available tests for Zika virus. By "commercially-available", I am not referring to a test you can buy at your local pharmacy like a pregnancy test. I am talking about the fact that most laboratories, even in the United States, don't yet have the capability to test for the virus.

The only places, so far, that have this ability are the Center for Disease Control and Prevention and several state laboratories. Testing must be requested from health authorities in the region to facilitate the process.

If a sample of blood serum can find its way to an appropriate laboratory for testing, Zika virus can be diagnosed by a study called "Reverse

Transcriptase-Polymerase Chain Reaction", or RT-PCR. This test identifies genetic material from Zika called "RNA". Antibodies formed by exposure to the virus might also be identified using an "IgM" test, but these antibodies could be confused with those of other viruses in the Flavivirus family such as Dengue. Telling these antibodies apart requires even another test (Plaque-Reduction Neutralization Testing or PRNT) that is also available only in advanced labs.

There are even more challenges physicians face other than just getting a sample of blood to a special lab. The Zika virus only spends a week or so in the blood (sometimes longer) during the acute illness; samples obtained for RT-PCR testing after that time may demonstrate no virus at all. The antibodies should still be present, however.

Another method of testing involves taking a sample of the amniotic fluid from the pregnant uterus. The amniotic fluid is the environment in which the fetus lives while it develops. This procedure is called "amniocentesis".

In amniocentesis, a needle is inserted through the abdomen and into the uterus. Ultrasound guidance is used to identify a pocket of fluid from which the sample is obtained. The fluid is then sent to the lab for Zika testing.

Today, amniocentesis is a safe procedure in experienced hands, but complications can still occur that might cause bleeding or injury to the fetus. It should only be used if head measurements are small or if there is evidence of Zika in the blood.

Given the widespread outbreaks, any baby born with microcephaly previously undetected by ultrasound should be tested for Zika virus, along with the mother.

The CDC has wisely chosen to make ZIKV a reportable disease. That is, local and state authorities must be notified every time a case is diagnosed. Until physicians realize the importance of reporting suspected cases, it will be impossible to know the true extent of the outbreak.

Microcephaly

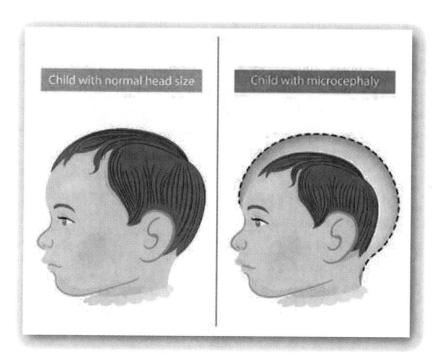

Child with normal head size | Child with microcephaly

The reason that Zika virus disease has made the news is not because of severe effects during the acute illness, but its potential to cause deformities in babies. Humans aren't perfect and don't produce perfect babies 100% of the time. One child with brain damage is a personal tragedy for the family, but an unusually large number of brain-damaged children can sorely test the ability of a nation, especially a poor one, to care for them.

Microcephaly is normally defined as a head circumference more than two standard deviations below the mean for age and sex. This correlates to the 2nd or 3rd percentile; that is, a smaller head than 97-98%

of newborns. Head measurements are standard components of obstetric ultrasound exams.

Microcephaly may occur alone or with other birth defects. Beside the possible connection with Zika virus, microcephaly is associated with genetic factors, exposure to toxins and drugs, and other infectious diseases. Excessive alcohol consumption has also been implicated. When infections like Rubella (German Measles) are the cause, the worst effects occur when exposed in the early part of the pregnancy. Other infections that are associated with microcephaly include:

* Varicella (Chicken Pox)
* Toxoplasmosis
* Cytomegalovirus
* Herpes Simplex
* Syphilis

It stands to reason that an infant with a greatly decreased head size would have a much smaller brain as well. A newborn may appear relatively normal at first, but develop a striking appearance as they grow. The head fails to grow in concert with nearby structures. That is, the face continues to develop but the cranium doesn't.

The result is a child with a small head and a receding forehead with loose skin on the scalp. Eyes may appear prominent. Intellectual milestones, such as speech, are also delayed or not reached at all. Other neurological effects such as seizures may be noted, as well as vision or hearing deficiencies.

Motor skills are often as delayed as intellectual development. The microcephalic child may be hyperactive and have issues with coordination. Severe cases may result in spastic muscles or even quadriplegia (partial paralysis). Short stature is commonly seen.

Not all infants born with microcephaly will be severely handicapped, and there appears to be a spectrum of effects all the way from minimal disability to incompatibility with life.

Other abnormalities that seem to be associated with Zika virus infection in the womb include intracranial calcifications. These calcifications might be visible on fetal ultrasound and may or may not be a consequence of the virus.

Treatment

As with many other viral infections, there is no known effective treatment for ZIKV. Antiviral drugs exist, for example, to treat influenza but these have no effect on members of the Flavivirus family. The anti-flu drug Oseltamivir (Tamiflu) decreases the severity and duration of the illness, but research is still ongoing for drugs that might have a beneficial effect on other viruses.

Therefore, treatment centers on alleviating the symptoms. Fever may be reduced with acetaminophen (Tylenol), which may also relieve pain in muscles and joints. Fluids should be given to prevent dehydration and the patient should be placed on bedrest until better.

Aspirin and NSAIDs such as ibuprofen should be avoided, as ZIKV may mimic its relative, Dengue Fever. Dengue Fever may affect the ability of a victim's blood to clot. Aspirin and NSAIDs may worsen the situation.

For the small number of victims that develop Guillain-Barre syndrome, certain therapies might lessen the severity of the signs and symptoms and hasten recovery.

Plasma exchange (also called plasmapheresis) and high-dose immunoglobulin therapy have been used and both are effective. Plasma exchange removes whole blood from the body and separates the red and white blood cells from the liquid part of the blood (also called "plasma"). The blood cells, but not the plasma, are then returned to the patient. The plasma is quickly replaced naturally. We don't know exactly why plasma exchange works, but it may be due to yet-undiscovered substances in the plasma.

Another option is immunoglobulin therapy. This method uses intravenous injections of proteins that the immune system uses to protect against invading organisms. Using high doses taken from, sometimes, thousands of normal donors, immunoglobulin therapy seems to lessen the damage to the nervous system. As with plasma exchange, researchers don't yet know how this works.

Although no specific treatment or cure against Zika virus is available as of this writing, a number of countries, including the United States, are working feverishly to produce a vaccine and drugs to deal with this virus. Estimates range from one to two years.

Perhaps the most effective way to control the spread of Zika virus is by prevention. Mosquito control programs are underway in many countries and will be discussed, along with other protective strategies, later in this book.

What the CDC Says

The Center for Disease Control and Prevention is the main arm of the government responsible for the protection of the health of the American public. When a new threat arises, the CDC must spring into action to place obstacles in the way of a new disease so that the homeland is shielded from its effects.

We look to the CDC for quick action, and that hasn't always been the case, as we saw during the Ebola epidemic of 2014. Eventually, however, protocols are set to combat the spread of infectious disease. Here are some statements that CDC director Tom Frieden made to CNN:

"Vaccines and antibiotics have made many infectious diseases a thing of the past; we've come to expect that public health and modern science can conquer all microbes. But nature is a formidable adversary. And Zika is our newest threat, particularly to pregnant women.

...At the Centers for Disease Control and Prevention -- where we identify, on average, one new health threat each year -- we work around the clock with an approach that prioritizes finding out what we need to know as fast as we can to protect Americans."

Dr. Frieden acknowledges our limitations, given the lack of research into Zika virus. The CDC can't predict the future, but it can work towards a better understanding of the challenge facing the United States. He writes: "Science doesn't have a crystal ball, but the CDC has great laboratories and the world's best disease detectives... CDC scientists as well as private companies are working to develop tests that can do this accurately. This is a priority, and we are working to do in weeks what would usually take months or years."

Across the Department of Health and Human Services, there is also important work related to Zika, particularly to speed the development of tests, treatments and vaccines.

Dr. Frieden promises that the CDC will have a "laser focus" when it comes to protecting the health and safety of U.S. citizens.

Now You Know: Now you know what the Zika virus is and how it has traveled to the Western Hemisphere and caused, possibly, millions of cases of infections. You learned about how the Zika virus is transmitted and a lot about the Aedes species of mosquitoes from egg to adult. You learned what the acute illness looks like, and that 80% of those infected have no symptoms at all.

You also now know about microcephaly, the birth defect that is causing so much concern in Brazil, and how it's identified. Lastly, you know how the presence of Zika virus in a person is confirmed using lab tests and the treatment options (or lack of them) that exist at present. You also know that the CDC recognizes the issue and has a plan of action is to combat the virus.

PART 2

Pandemic Disease

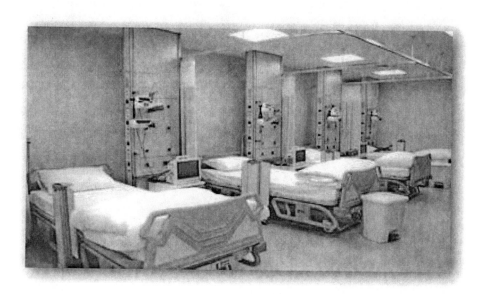

IN MODERN TIMES, WE HAVE become highly dependent on the high technology that has, in many cases, eliminated the scourge of infectious disease. Antibiotic and antiviral medications are now available in their 3rd or 4th generation, and physicians aren't reluctant to use them when necessary. Yet, recent history tells us that infectious agents, especially viruses, can get out of control.

Officially, an infection is defined as the invasion by, and multiplication of, a microscopic organism known as a "pathogen". A pathogen is any agent that can cause a disease. Pathogens cause injury to tissues by producing toxins that cause damage in various ways. Not every microbe is a pathogen; in fact, some are beneficial or even necessary for human life. A good example is the bacteria that lives in your intestinal tract.

Pathogens are often carried by "vectors", from the latin word *vectus, "one who carries"*. These are microbes, animals or persons that carry and transmit a disease to others. These vectors may or may not be ill themselves: A mosquito, for example, carries the organism that causes Zika in humans but doesn't experience the disease. "Typhoid Mary" was a domestic servant and cook that carried that epidemic disease to many other people without having physical signs of it herself. The elimination of a vector from the environment (terminating Mary's employment, for example) usually leads to cessation of the spread of the disease.

Bacteria, Viruses, and Protozoa

To understand infectious diseases, we must first know a little about the organisms that cause them. The main pathogens you'll see are bacteria, viruses, and protozoa.

Bacteria are single-celled organisms that were among the first life forms to appear on Earth, and are present almost everywhere. Scientists are even searching for signs of bacteria on the planet Mars. Bacteria inhabit soil, water, and even your body.

There are typically 40 million bacteria in a gram of soil and a million bacteria in a milliliter of water. If you took into account the entire population of bacteria on Earth, their mass would exceed that of all plants and animals on the planet. When bacteria reach a certain size, they reproduce by splitting in two, a process called binary fission.

Most bacteria are beneficial; you wouldn't be able to digest food with them, and they even live on your skin. Some, however, are pathogens and cause infectious diseases, including:

* Cholera
* Anthrax
* The bubonic plague

* Leprosy
* Tuberculosis
* Typhoid Fever
* Strep throat

The most common fatal bacterial diseases affect the lungs, with tuberculosis alone killing about 2 million people a year, mostly in underdeveloped countries.

Rickettsia differ from other bacteria in that their survival depends on entry, growth, and reproduction within a host cell. Rickettsiae are the cause of typhus, Rocky Mountain Spotted fever, and a number of other infectious diseases. *Rickettsia* do not, however, cause rickets, a deformity of long bones which is a result of vitamin D deficiency.

Bacteria can be killed by the use of antibiotics.

Viruses are microscopic infectious agents that can reproduce only inside the living cells of other organisms. Viral particles on their own are known as virions, which only act as a living organism when they enter a host cell. Viruses can infect all types of life forms, from animals and plants all the way down to bacteria.

Examples of common human diseases caused by viruses include:

* Influenza
* Chicken Pox
* Measles
* Rabies

- Hepatitis
- HIV
- Ebola
- Zika
- The common cold

Viruses spread in many ways: Zika is transmitted, for example, by mosquitoes. Influenza viruses are spread by coughing and sneezing. Intestinal viruses are transmitted by the anal–oral route and are passed from person to person by close contact or may enter the body in food or water. HIV is one of several viruses transmitted through sexual contact. Zika has also been shown to occasionally be spread in this manner.

Viral infections provoke an immune response in your body that usually kills the infecting virus. Immune responses to viruses can also be produced by vaccines, which confer an immunity to the specific viral infection. However, some viruses, including those that cause AIDS and viral hepatitis, evade these immune responses and can result in chronic illness.

Antibiotics have no effect on viruses, but there are a number of antiviral drugs that can treat certain illnesses like influenza.

Protozoa are one-celled microbes with animal-like behavior, such as the ability to move. They are restricted to moist or aquatic environments. Amoebas are a form of protozoa. Protozoa can cause infectious diseases in humans:

- Malaria
- Giardia

* Dysentery
* Sleeping Sickness
* Amoebiasis

Some protozoa can be killed with antibiotics; others require more specialized medicines.

Pandemic vs. Epidemic vs. Endemic

You have probably heard about epidemics and pandemics, but what are they? What's the difference between them, and how do they differ from a disease that's "endemic"?

An **endemic** disease is one that's regularly found among particular people or in a certain area. Obesity, for example, is endemic in the United States; Malaria is endemic in many tropical countries.

An **epidemic** is a rapid widespread occurrence of an infectious disease in a community that isn't always seen there. Swine flu, for example, is an epidemic disease not constantly seen in an area.

A **pandemic** occurs when an infectious disease runs rampant throughout a large region or, in the case of the Great Spanish Flu Epidemic of 1918, the entire world.

How does an epidemic reach pandemic status? The World Health Organization rates its level of concern about a disease entering a new area with "Phase" alerts. These go as follows:

Phase 1: A virus is found in animals; no known infections in humans.

Phase 2: The disease has caused proven infection in humans.

Joseph Alton, MD

Phase 3: Small clusters of disease occur in humans but do not affect entire communities.

Phase 4: The disease now affects entire communities. The disease qualifies as an epidemic, but the risk for a pandemic, although greatly increased, is unlikely.

Phase 5: Spread of disease between humans is occurring in more than one country in a region. The Ebola outbreak of 2014 is an example of this phase, with communities affected in several different bordering West African countries.

Phase 6: Community-wide outbreaks are in at least one additional country in different regions. Although Ebola failed to reach this phase, both Zika and Chikungunya virus did and carry the title of full-blown pandemic.

Understanding Immunity

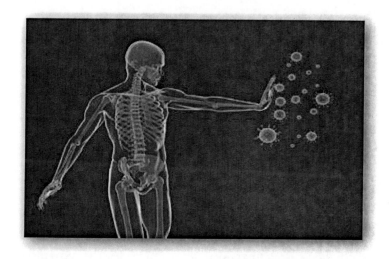

Mosquitoes that carry Zika virus don't get sick from it. It has no effect on their health as they carry and transmit it to humans. As such, we can say that they are "immune" to the ill effects of the disease.

Immunity is the ability of your immune system to resist a particular infection or toxin. This can refer to resistance of an entire species (humans, for example, don't get fish diseases like fin rot) or the resistance of a particular individual to an illness (Typhoid Mary, for example, carried the typhoid germ without getting sick herself). Immunity is affected by many factors, such as age, genetics, and stress from chronic illness or nutritional and environmental factors.

There are several types of immunity. They are:

SHORT-TERM IMMUNITY

When an infectious agent is detected, the body responds by producing an immune response which attacks the invader. During an epidemic, the human population's ability to generate an immune defense increases its resistance to the disease. It is this property of the human body that causes the epidemic to eventually collapse.

LONG-TERM IMMUNITY

The body's defenses retain a type of 'memory' of the offending organism. If the pathogen returns to the area, that memory causes the body to produce a faster and stronger response against it. This is especially true with viral infections, often giving lifetime protection. An example would be "Varicella", a viral illness otherwise known as 'chicken pox". Once you have had chicken pox, you are usually immune for the remainder of your life. The current thinking is that the same can be said for Zika virus.

NATURAL IMMUNITY

A particular individual, or occasionally an entire segment of the population, might possess the ability to resist a pathogen due to genetic "memory" passed on from generation to generation.

The Native American populace of the New World had an extraordinarily high mortality rate when exposed to smallpox by the first European explorers. Those same explorers, however, had a much higher survival rate due to natural immunity conferred on them by their ancestors' centuries of previous exposures.

HERD IMMUNITY

When a large group (a "herd") possesses immunity, non-immune individuals within it enjoy a certain protection due to fewer exposures to an infection that may otherwise be fatal to them. The most common example today relates to vaccinated populations. If an unvaccinated person moves into an area where many are immune due to vaccinations, their likelihood of exposure to the disease drops significantly.

The immune "herd" confers a certain level of protection to the non-immune by lowering their chance of ever being exposed to the disease. If many unvaccinated people move into an area, however, the overall "herd immunity" may be lost. This situation is thought to be the cause for the resurgence of Measles in some places.

History of Pandemic Disease

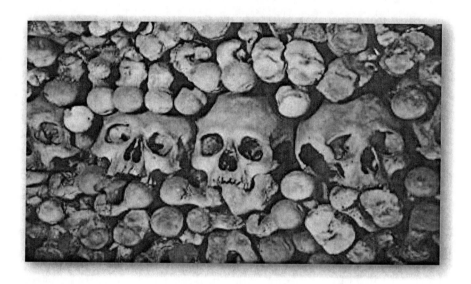

You might consider pandemics to be a once in a lifetime event, but two of them, Zika and Chikungunya virus, have occurred in successive years. Indeed, pandemics have occurred throughout history with 3 or 4 serious ones identified every century. Some of the most devastating pandemics have changed the course of history. They include:

The Antonine Plague: Named for Roman Emperor and philosopher Marcus Aurelius Antoninus, the outbreak began in 165 AD and lasted 15 years. An estimated five million people died from what is now thought to have been smallpox. It was believed to have begun in Mesopotamia (modern-day Iraq) and spread all the way to Rome with returning soldiers. At one point during the extended pandemic, an estimated 2,000 Romans died each day. This wasn't a plague that only hit the poor. Marcus Aurelius himself is thought to have been one of the victims.

The Plague of Justinian: In the year 541, rats from Egyptian grain boats brought a pestilence to the Eastern Roman Empire that would ultimately leave approximately 25 million people dead. Even the emperor himself (Justinian I, for whom the plague was named) got the disease, although he survived. As many as 5,000 people died per day in the capital city of Constantinople. Before it was over, about 40 percent of the city's population was dead—so many and so quickly that bodies were left unburied in piles. The entire Mediterranean coast lost about a quarter of its population. Modern experts now believe that the outbreak was the first recorded case of the bubonic plague.

The Black Death: The middle ages were wracked with waves of bubonic plague pandemics, which was by then known as the Black Death, for the color of lumps, called buboes, in the armpits and groins of the victims. It was so devastating that most of us have heard of it, although it's been hundreds of years since the last major pandemic of the disease. Another form of the plague, the pneumonic plague, was so deadly that it was said that you could get it in the morning and be dead by nightfall.

Infected sailors from Asia arrived in Sicily around the middle of the 14th century, and from 1347 to 1351, the Black Death depopulated Europe and most of the world. 75-150 million deaths are attributed to it, at a time when there were about 450 million people total on the planet. Half of Europe died in a span of only four years.

The Spanish Flu of 1918: As the First World War was grinding to a close, a new strain of influenza began to appear simultaneously in multiple countries around the world. The disease spread quickly due to the poor sanitary conditions in places where troops were fighting. It was named The Spanish Flu (despite the fact that it didn't actually come from Spain). The pandemic burned out quickly in late 1919 for unknown reasons, but not before it killed anywhere from 50 to 100 million people, half of which died within the first few months of the outbreak.

HIV/AIDS: Due to a virus that attacks the immune system, Human Immunodeficiency Virus, also known as HIV, appeared in the early 1980s. In many cases, the infection led to Acquired Immunodeficiency Syndrome, also called AIDS. While medicine has made great strides in dealing with this disease in developed countries, it is still raging in many parts of Africa. Over 30 years, at least 60 million people had been infected by AIDS and 25 million have died. In 2008 an estimated 1.2 million Americans had HIV, but Sub-Saharan Africa alone was home to 22.9 million cases, with one in five adults infected. About 35.3 million people were believed to have HIV in a study performed in 2012.

Many other diseases have reached epidemic and pandemic status over the years. Cholera, a diarrheal disease, was first seen in India and has since caused 3-5 million cases a year and millions of deaths over time, even though antibiotics will cure the disease. It was especially widespread in Haiti after the devastating earthquake in that country some years ago. Diseases like Measles, Tuberculosis, Typhus, Smallpox, and even Syphilis have caused widespread outbreaks at one point or another in time.

How Pandemics Spread

A pandemic isn't a pandemic, by definition, unless it spreads. We touched upon how Zika virus is spread by mosquitoes and by sexual contact, but more research is needed to rule out other methods of transmission. Here are some ways that pandemic disease cause community-wide outbreaks:

Ingestion - Eating infected animals is a common cause for the viruses to spread in humans. Bats and monkeys are part of the diet of many people in Africa, and are known carriers of the Ebola virus. Working with poultry is thought to be a reason that humans get the bird flu.

Inhalation - Spread through air or by breathing in droplets from the infected, such as blood splatter, phlegm, or saliva. Bodily fluids usually have a great deal of bacteria or viruses and some of them can be aerosolized into the air. Influenza is a typical example. Blood and phlegm will, if they enter your mouth, nose, eyes, or an open cut or sore, easily pass their germs to a new host.

Injection – From needle sticks or other medical items. Hepatitis is a disease commonly passed this way, but almost any disease is a candidate for spread in this manner. It could be argued that a mosquito "injects" Zika virus into a human.

Absorption - Touching secretions from the infections and then touching mouth, eyes, or open sores. This happens more often than you might imagine. Just look at the average person for a while and count the number of times they touch their face. The West African cultural practice of family members personally washing the body of deceased Ebola victims is probably responsible for entire families wiped out by the disease.

Sexual - From the semen and bodily secretions of infected persons. Syphilis is a disease commonly sexually transmitted and, from the 1400s to the early 1900s, was a scourge of almost every civilized country. Ebola can be transmitted sexually for weeks after a patient has recovered from the disease. So far, several cases of ZIKV has been shown to have spread by sexual contact.

Pregnancy – Passed from mother to fetus – ZIKV, HIV, Syphilis, and Ebola are just some of the diseases that can be passed this way.

If bodily fluids from sexual contact can pass Zika from human to human, it stands to reason that other bodily fluid will, also. As we learn more, many of the above methods of transmission not currently ascribed to the virus will probably be added to the list of possible ways to spread it.

There is one more way that pandemic diseases can be spread: by complacency. Lack of attention to infection control in high-risk areas is probably the most likely reason for the spread of an infection. In the countries affected by Zika virus, the failure to aggressively control mosquito populations is the cause for its explosive spread.

Candidates for the Next Pandemic

Zika virus is the current pandemic, following the Chikungunya virus from the previous year. Both have serious consequences: Zika has tragic effects on newborns, and Chikungunya causes long-standing and debilitating joint pain in many of its victims. Neither ZIKV nor Chikungunya is particularly lethal, however; most sufferers go through a flu-like illness and then recover fully.

As you saw in our review of the history of pandemics, not all outbreaks of infectious diseases will have low mortality rates. This section will outline a list of possible pandemics that could arrive in the uncertain future in the form of viruses, bacteria, and protozoa.

VIRAL PANDEMIC DISEASES

Influenza: Influenza, or "the flu", is by far the most common viral disease associated with the word "pandemic". Indeed, perhaps 5% of the world's population gets it every year. Sometimes it's mild and sometimes it's severe, but at least 250,000 people will die each year with influenza listed as a factor on their death certificate. In pandemic years, the number rises to the millions.

Major flu pandemics occur a few times each century. We mentioned the worst one, the Spanish Flu of 1918-9, previously. The most recent one was the Swine Flu pandemic of 2009-10: There were 60 million cases, but only about 12,500 deaths in the U.S.

Influenzas are categorized by the "Ha Na" system. Influenza A viruses (the most common) are divided into subtypes based upon the nature of certain proteins that exist on their surface. These are called *Hemaglutinins (Ha)* and *Neuraminidases (Na)*. There are 18 different hemaglutinins and 11 neuraminidases which have been identified so far, with more discovered every year. Your immunity against one virus subtype does not necessarily work against another.

The most common symptoms of influenza are:

* Fever and Chills
* Cough
* Headache
* Muscle Ache
* Fatigue

Sore throat and nasal congestion may occur but are more commonly seen in the common cold. Colds are caused by different viruses than influenza.

Influenza is an "airborne" illness. This means that it is transmitted through the air by coughs or sneezes. Influenza can also be transmitted by direct contact with nasal secretions, or through contact with contaminated surfaces. Luckily, influenza viruses can be inactivated by sunlight, disinfectants, and detergents.

Treatment of influenza revolves around treating the individual symptoms, although the antiviral drug Oseltamivir (Tamiflu) and some others are effective if started within the first 48 hours of symptoms. Other treatments that are useful include:

- Fever reducers (acetaminophen, ibuprofen)
- Pain relief (acetaminophen, ibuprofen)
- Decongestants (pseudoephrine, etc.)
- Anti-Diarrheals (loperamide)
- Vitamins and natural immune boosters
- Oral rehydration Solutions (Gatorade, Pedialyte)

Rehydration solutions contain electrolytes. An electrolyte most commonly refers to salts or ions in the blood that carry a charge. These substances are essential to various bodily functions and must be in balance to stay healthy.

Oral rehydration solution can actually be made at home. To produce your own rehydration solution: Add...

- 6-8 teaspoons of sugar to a liter of clean water (2 liters for children).
- 1 teaspoon salt/liter (sodium chloride).
- 1/4-1/2 teaspoon salt subsitute, a product in your local supermarket for those who can't have salt but like the taste of it. Salt substitute adds potassium, an important electrolyte, to the solution.
- 1/4 teaspoon baking soda/liter (bicarbonate).

Vaccinations against influenza are usually made available to people in developed countries in an effort to confer immunity to the populace. They are given before the expected arrival of the virus. Vaccines are most effective if the flu virus is similar to last year's strain. This is because they use components of that virus to produce this year's vaccine.

If the virus has mutated significantly, the vaccine may be ineffective. Ordinarily, flu vaccine is 60 to 70% effective in preventing the disease. In one recent year, however, it only conferred 19% protection.

Ebola: The last epidemic disease to receive widespread attention from the media was the Ebola virus. Although it never caused community-wide outbreaks on different continents (thus, never reaching pandemic status), its high death rate of close to 50% caused great alarm before it finally came under control.

To get an idea of the lethality of Ebola, the Spanish Flu pandemic of 1918-9 had a 2% death rate. If Ebola had spread as far and wide as the Spanish Flu, entire countries might have been depopulated.

The Ebola virus is one of three members of the Filoviridae virus family. Ebola was first reported in 1976 in the Democratic Republic of Congo. It's named after the river where the first victims were identified. There are several known varieties of the virus, which suggests that it has mutated a number of times.

Most viruses in the Filoviridae family cause "hemorrhagic fevers". These can kill in several ways: internal bleeding, organ failure, and/or severe dehydration. After an incubation period of 2-21 days, the disease results in a massive viremia (large viral concentrations in the blood) that damages the cells that form blood vessels. As the disease progresses, a percentage of cases develop uncontrolled bleeding leads to extreme fluid loss and can cause hypotensive shock. Most deaths occur, not from hemorrhage, but from organ failure and dehydration.

Ebola is "zoonotic," which means that it passes between animals and humans. The main reservoir is thought to be fruit bats, but it has been found in gorillas, monkeys, forest antelope, chimpanzees, and even porcupines. Zika virus requires a mosquito to pass it along, but it doesn't appear to have an animal population that regularly passes the virus on to humans.

Humans and apes can get the disease by coming into close contact with the body or bodily fluids (blood, vomit, mucus, droppings, etc.) of an infected animal. Other animals (say, an antelope) can get it by eating grass that has bat droppings on it. It's thought that the 2014 outbreak in West Africa began when some villagers ate incompletely-cooked fruit bats.

Once the virus spreads to a human, person-to-person transmission is possible, even likely if there is close contact. With ZIKV, however, person to person transmission has been rarely documented, at least at present.

MERS: MERS stands for Middle East Respiratory Syndrome. MERS is caused by a coronavirus called MERS-CoV. MERS originated in the Middle East and has been linked to respiratory disease in camels: A recent study reports that 75% of camels in the area have evidence of past exposure to the virus. MERS appears to be most commonly transmitted through air droplets.

Once infected with Middle East Respiratory Syndrome, the patient begins to show signs of the disease in 10-12 days. Symptoms of MERS-CoV infection include fever, productive cough, nasal congestion, and shortness of breath. Some cases present with gastrointestinal symptoms like nausea, vomiting, and diarrhea. If the patient worsens, pneumonia (an infection of the lung) and organ failure occurs. The disease carries with it a 30% death rate, even higher in the most recent outbreak in South Korea that originated with a worker from the Middle East.

SARS: SARS stands for Sudden Acute Respiratory Syndrome; it is a coronavirus related to MERS and was found in certain parts of Asia a decade ago. It was characterized by sudden onset of high fever, headache, cough, and occasionally, diarrhea. The mortality from SARS-CoV is about 10%. There have been no outbreaks since 2003.

Measles: Measles is a highly contagious airborne virus that was once so common it was considered a childhood rite of passage. The disease is so infectious that there is a 90% chance of contracting the illness if an unvaccinated person is exposed to it. The disease was almost eradicated in the U.S. in the 2000's, but has experienced a resurgence due to resistance on the part of some to vaccination. In some areas of the United States, 1 in 8 children are not vaccinated.

Also known as **Rubeola**, Measles shouldn't be confused with **Rubella** (German Measles) or **Roseola**, a milder viral illness also seen in childhood. Millions of cases are reported each year worldwide, with 135,000 deaths in 2011. In the U.S., numbers have been as low as 37 in a year. In 2014, however, 610 U.S. cases were reported, and outbreaks can be expected in the future as "herd" immunity breaks down in communities with large numbers of unvaccinated children.

Measles patients present, usually, with a fever as high as 104 degrees Fahrenheit. 2-3 days later, a red patchy rash appears, usually starting on the head and face and then working its way downward, similar to Zika virus. In Measles, however, so many "spots" develop that the patches coalesce into even bigger blotches as times goes on. Other symptoms often resemble respiratory and eye infections. You may see the "**three C's**":

* **C**ough
* **C**oryza (head cold symptoms like nasal congestion, etc.)
* **C**onjunctivits (Pink Eye)

Mosquito borne viruses: Mosquito-borne viruses like Zika are found everywhere from St. Louis to the Japanese mainland. More and more cases are found every year in new areas, causing damage to a number of organ systems, from the nervous system to the intestinal tract. Some viruses related to ZikV have run rampant among wide areas, including:

* Yellow Fever
* Dengue Fever
* Chikungunya Virus
* West Nile Virus

Most of these viruses begin with flu-like symptoms, but progress to causing various serious medical problems such as bleeding disorders, joint infections, and even brain inflammation, depending on which virus is involved.

Yellow fever took a major toll on workers during the construction of the Panama Canal. Dengue Fever was common among soldiers in combat zones during World War II. Chikungunya caused the most cases of mosquito-borne viral illness in the last few years when it crossed the Atlantic in 2014. It's thought that some countries, like the Domincan Republic, suffered economically due to lost work days due to the illness. In all, one to two million Chikungunya cases were reported. More information about these mosquito-borne illnesses can be found later in this book.

BACTERIAL PANDEMIC DISEASES

Although the above-listed diseases are all caused by viruses, bacteria are still the cause of many epidemics despite the availability of effective antibiotics. This often occurs due to contamination of food and water, but some are transmissible through the air.

The Plague: Plague, also known as the "Black Death", is the disease perhaps most commonly associated with pandemics in the mind of the public.. Plague is caused by the bacteria Yersinia Pestis, found in fleas that infest rats. Different forms of plague can be spread in the air, by direct contact, or by contaminated water or improperly prepared food.

The symptoms of plague depend on the concentrated areas of infection in each person: bubonic plague infects lymph nodes causing accumulation of bacteria, blood, and pus called "buboes" in the groin and armpits, pneumonic plague infects the lungs, and septicemic plague occurs when the bacteria hits the bloodstream. Isolated cases of plague are still reported every year in various parts of the world, including the United States.

Infection in a human occurs when bitten by a flea that has itself been infected by biting a rodent that carries the disease. The bacteria multiply inside the flea, sticking together to form a plug that blocks its stomach and causes it to starve. Despite this, the flea continues to feed on the host, vomiting the blood tainted with the bacteria back into the bite wound. Thus, the plague infects new victims as the dying flea travels from host to host.

Of the various types of plague, pneumonic plague does damage the fastest and kills almost all infected in 1 or 2 days if untreated. Despite this, the disease is treatable with antibiotics such as doxycycline, tetracycline, or ciprofloxacin, if detected very early.

Tuberculosis: Tuberculosis (TB) was once called "Consumption", as it gave the victim the appearance of being consumed by the disease. It is an infection caused by a type of bacteria called *Mycobacteria tuberculosis*. Tuberculosis typically attacks the lungs, but can also affect other parts of the body, even female internal organs.

It is spread through the air when people who have active TB cough, sneeze, or otherwise expel respiratory fluids. Most infections don't have symptoms. I, myself, have tested positive for this disease, thanks to my work with Cuban refugees during the Mariel boatlift in 1980.

Once in the body, TB is sometimes walled off by the immune system. It can, however, eventually progress to active disease years later, especially in malnourished or weakened victims.

One-third of the world's population is thought to have been infected with *M. tuberculosis*. It is so common that entire hospitals devoted to the disease, called sanitariums, still exist in some countries.

Although TB can be treated with long-term therapy using a combination of antibiotics, some cases have proven to be totally resistant.

Cholera: Cholera, caused by a bacterium called *Vibrio cholera*, has been an epidemic disease in many countries over the centuries, with a recent severe outbreak in Haiti after the earthquake there some years ago. It is transmitted through contaminated food and water. An estimated 3-5 million cases and over 100,000 deaths occur each year around the world.

Cholera is a diarrheal disease. In extreme cases, patients may lose over one quart of fluid per hour and up to 3-5 gallons of watery bowel movements a day. Additional symptoms include nausea and vomiting, abdominal pain, and fever. Cholera leads to severe dehydration, which will cause rapid organ failure if fluids are not replaced. Several antibiotics are effective against it, including doxycycline, ciprofloxacin, and azithromycin.

Typhus: Typhus is another epidemic disease found in unhygienic conditions. It's passed by rickettsial germs that are found in fleas on rats, similar to plague. High fever, cough, rashes, headaches, joint and muscle pain are just some of the symptoms found in the two different types of this disease. Doxycycline will cure the disease if treated early.

Typhoid Fever: So named because it appears much like Typhus, Typhoid is a bacterial disease transmitted by the ingestion of food or water contaminated with a microbe called Salmonella. The patient often develops a rash known as "rose spots" with high fevers and other symptoms. The infection can travel, in stages, to various organs such as the liver and cause bleeding or even perforations in the intestine. Luckily, it can be treated with various antibiotics such as ciprofloxacin.

PROTOZOAL PANDEMIC DISEASES

As if viruses and bacteria weren't enough, protozoa are also the culprits in some pandemic and epidemic diseases. Protozoa are one-celled microbes that can move using tail-like appendages called "flagella". They are restricted to moist or aquatic environments.

Malaria: Malaria is a mosquito-borne infectious disease of humans and other animals caused by parasitic protozoans called plasmodia. The classic symptom of malaria is "paroxysm", a cyclical occurrence of sudden coldness followed by shivering and then fever and sweating. Episodes begin after an incubation period usually lasting 10 days to 4 weeks. These paroxysms can occur every two or three days and return more and more frequently in untreated cases. This leads to eventual damage to multiple organ systems.

Malaria is endemic in almost every tropical or sub-tropical country. The World Health Organization estimates that in 2012, there were 207 million cases of malaria. That year, the disease is estimated to have killed between 473,000 and 789,000 people, many of whom were children in Africa.

There are some natural treatments for Malaria still in use today. One is Quinine, which occurs naturally in the bark of the cinchona tree. Quinine is a component of the common drink mixer tonic water. Quinine sulfate is commercially available under the brand name Qualaquin; *Artemisia Annua* is a plant from which the antimalarial drug Artemisinin is derived and considered an effective therapy.

Amebiasis: Amebiasis is an infection with a microbe called *Entamoeba histolytica*. It is usually passed in improperly prepared food or by contact associated with poor toilet hygiene. Amebiasis causes a bloody mucus diarrhea known as dysentery. It is estimated that about 40,000 to 100,000 people worldwide die annually from the disease, but many more are asymptomatic carriers. The infection can sometimes last for years if untreated. Metronidazole is the antibiotic agent of choice.

Giardiasis: Giardiasis is a parasitic disease caused by the protozoan *Giardia lamblia*. It is the most common disease-causing parasitic infection in humans worldwide; in 2013, there were estimated to be about 280 million people worldwide with symptomatic giardiasis.

Besides humans, the organism inhabits the digestive tract of a wide variety of domestic and wild animal species. Symptoms include loss of appetite, diarrhea, loose or watery stools, stomach cramps, and upset stomach. Bloating and burping is sometimes seen due to excessive gas. Contaminated water is thought to be the most like cause of the illness. Like Amebiasis, metronidazole is an effective drug to eliminate the infection.

All of the viruses, bacteria, and protozoa described in this section are still candidates for the next epidemic. A few of history's pandemics are no longer considered an issue. This is, of course, unless a major disaster occurs that eliminates access to modern medical care. Two viral diseases, in particular, should be mentioned here: Smallpox and Polio:

Smallpox: Smallpox is caused by infection with the Variola virus. It's characterized by the rapid onset of high fevers, followed by a rash in which many dimpled blisters called pustules appear, first in the oral cavity, and then all over the body. It's closely related to Varicella, also called "chickenpox". Smallpox, however, affects the palms of the hands and the soles of the feet, while chickenpox does not. Additionally, chickenpox pustules are of varying sizes, while smallpox pustules are all very nearly the same size.

Once inhaled, the virus spreads quickly and can kill, especially in populations that have never been exposed to it, such as the natives of the New World during the Age of Discovery. The disease was deadly enough in the Old World, as well, where it killed an estimated 400,000 Europeans annually during the closing years of the 18th century, including a number of kings and queens. George Washington is a famous survivor of the disease.

Smallpox is well known for causing scarring, and sometimes blindness if the scars are on the eyes. Of all those infected, 20–60% (and over 80% of infected children) died from the disease. Worldwide vaccination programs have led to it eradication; the last naturally-occurring case was in 1977.

Polio: Officially called "Poliomyelitis", Polio is a debilitating disease caused by the Poliovirus. Anal-oral contamination due to poor hand hygiene can transmit the highly contagious virus. The incubation period is usually 6-20 days. The disease presents with a wide range of symptoms and severity; indeed, some people experience no symptoms at all.

Polio can cause symptoms like fever, sore throat, and nausea. Although symptomatic cases resolve within a short time, the virus enters the nervous system in a small percentage of cases. In these patients, muscle weakness and paralysis occurs, which is sometimes permanent. As a result of the number of children affected, Polio was also known as "infantile paralysis".

Epidemics of Polio occurred in Europe and the United States throughout the late 19th and early to mid-20th centuries. As a result of vaccines developed in the 1950s, however, Polio became rare, and there is hope of complete eradication by 2018. There were 98 cases reported worldwide in 2015, some in the war-torn Middle East.

Mosquito-Borne Viruses Related to Zika

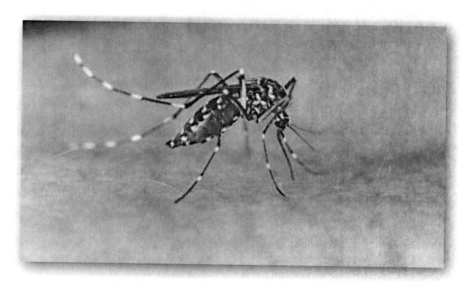

Due to its ability to spread disease, the mosquito is the most dangerous creature on the planet. Besides the worldwide presence of Malaria, mosquito-borne Flaviviruses like Zika are found everywhere from St. Louis to Japan. This family of viruses causes damage to a number of organ systems, from the nervous system to the intestinal tract.

Some viruses related to ZIKV have run rampant among wide areas, including:

* Dengue Fever
* Yellow Fever

* Chikungunya Virus
* West Nile Virus
* St. Louis Encephalitis
* Japanese Encephalitis
* Murray Valley Encephalitis

Most of these viruses begin with flu-like symptoms, but may progress, depending on the infection, to bleeding disorders, joint infections, and even brain inflammation.

Yellow Fever: Yellow fever is a type of equatorial hemorrhagic fever well-known historically for its toll on workers during the construction of the Panama Canal. It is found in two forms: urban and jungle. The jungle form, as you might imagine, is the original and was transmitted by forest mosquitoes to non-human primates. The urban version affects man and is transmitted through the Aedes mosquito.

After an incubation period of 3-6 days, fever, chills, muscle aches, and headaches occur along with nausea and vomiting. Like Zika, conjunctivitis (inflammation of the whites of the eyes) may occur. Most recover in a few days.

The more severe cases, however, will see the onset of jaundice, a yellowing of the skin due to liver malfunction that gives Yellow Fever its name. Bleeding disorders begin to cause spontaneous hemorrhage from nose, gums, and the intestinal tract. Once this point is reached, a 50% death rate is expected. An effective vaccine has been available since 1937.

Dengue Fever: Dengue is another hemorrhagic fever in the Flavivus family. Hundreds of thousands of cases are reported annually in tropical and subtropical areas throughout the planet. Dengue is a prevalent public health problem in Southeast Asia, the Caribbean, Central America, North America, South America, and Africa.

Dengue, like many mosquito-borne illnesses, is not transmitted directly from person to person. In some areas, however, the mosquito population is so large that 50% of people are infected. The highest number of cases occur during periods of highest rainfall and temperatures, when *Aedes aegypti* is most numerous.

Initial symptoms include fever, severe headache, muscle and joint pain, rashes, and pain behind the eyes. Severe cases are characterized by fever, abdominal pain, and bleeding disorders. These symptoms, if left untreated, lead to life-threatening organ collapse, mostly in children. There is no vaccine available at present.

Chikungunya: Due to the devotion of media attention given the Ebola epidemic in West Africa in 2014, Chikungunya was hardly noticed when it first crossed the Atlantic. This mosquito-borne virus, however, caused almost 2 million cases during its run and still exists in tropical South America and the Caribbean. Hospitalizations were so common due to the severity of the symptoms that it's thought that some countries, like the Domincan Republic, suffered economically due to lost work days.

Chikungunya (an African term meaning "that which bends up") is a viral illness that is not fatal, but causes excruciating pain in joints as well as a high fever. The pain is reminiscent of severe arthritis and can last for weeks, months, or even years. Other symptoms, besides joint pain and fever, include:

* Headache
* Nausea and vomiting
* Red eyes
* Sensitivity to light
* Leg swelling

We don't yet know what causes some of the above symptoms. Although previously unheard-of, the virus isn't brand new; it was first originally identified in 1952, but is thought, in hindsight, to have caused outbreaks since the 18th century. Epidemics of Chikungunya overseas have been reported in regions of the Indian Ocean, Africa, Asia, and some Pacific Islands.

Monkeys and apes were original reservoirs of the virus, but it is thought to have traveled to this hemisphere through rats and other rodents. Since it was new to the area, few were immune, causing the number of cases to skyrocket.

West Nile virus: West Nile fever is a dengue-like illness that occurs in Africa, Asia, and the Mediterranean. Most of the adult populations of Egypt and Iran have been exposed, according to antibody tests. Unlike some other Flaviviruses, West Nile is transmitted by Culex mosquito species as opposed to Aedes.

Children will usually only experience a mild febrile illness with a rash. Adults may experience a dengue-like illness which includes headache, muscle aches, joint pains, vomiting, diarrhea, and rash. Most people with West Nile virus disease recover completely, but fatigue and weakness can last for weeks or months. The elderly may develop an inflammation of the brain called "encephalitis" which is sometimes fatal. No vaccine for the virus is currently available.

St. Louis encephalitis: The most important endemic flavivirus in North America (so far) is St. Louis encephalitis. It occurs throughout the Americas. It is closely related to Japanese encephalitis and the Murray Valley encephalitis viruses. Thousands of cases of St. Louis encephalitis have been documented over a period of years. The virus is maintained in nature by a bird-mosquito-bird cycle.

Those infected often don't complain of symptoms, but when they do, there are three levels of severity. Headaches and fever are the mildest but can progress to an inflammation of the lining of the spinal cord (aseptic meningitis). Inflammation of the brain (encephalitis) is the most dangerous consequence.

Japanese encephalitis: You won't hear much about Japanese encephalitis (JE), but there are nearly 68000 cases each year, with 15000-20000 deaths. JE mostly affects children. After a mild flu-like stage, the disease progresses in some cases to the brain and kills 20-50% of those that reach that stage.

A vaccine to prevent Japanese encephalitis has been in use for years, but cases are still found in India, Asia, and the Pacific Islands. A closely related viral disease, Murray Valley encephalitis, is found in Australia and New Guinea.

It should be noted that the majority of people infected with the above viruses have no symptoms at all. Although this isn't a bad thing, it can make diagnosis difficult and obstruct the efforts of scientists to determine infection rates and the true geographic distribution.

Care for the Pandemic Patient

Today, we have modern medical facilities and advanced techniques to isolate a sick patient from healthy people. In a true pandemic scenario, however, medical facilities might be overwhelmed and the head of household may have to become the main caregiver. Although the home won't have advanced medical equipment, the family "medic" can still put together an environment that will speed the recovery of those infected while keeping the rest safe.

Many think that a pandemic will throw us back to an earlier age, medically, but we have the benefit of all the knowledge gained since then. The concepts of how contagious disease is spread and how to maintain an effective "sick room" will greatly increase survival rates over those seen in previous eras.

Sick rooms for infectious diseases must be planned carefully to achieve the best result. Choose a place at one end of the house away from common areas such as the kitchen or living room. This area should be well-ventilated with windows to let in fresh air and light. Despite this, the room should have a door that can be closed or other barrier.

If power is not an issue, you'll probably have air conditioning. In this instance, the air ducts should be covered with sheeting or duct tape to prevent airborne viruses to make their way to the rest of the house.

Furnishings should be minimal, with a work surface, an exam area, and bed spaces. Sofas and chairs upholstered with fabric can harbor pathogens (disease-causing organisms) and should be avoided if possible. The floor should be bare of carpeting, as well. Even bedding for the contagious might best be covered in plastic. The more areas that can be wiped down and disinfected easily, the better.

A simple disinfectant solution is necessary for cleaning purposes and can be made inexpensively. Household bleach is an excellent choice. A 10% bleach solution can be used on a daily basis to wipe down contaminated surfaces.

To prepare a bleach solution, you'll need:

* A mixing container that can hold ten measures or on which you mark ten equal increments.
* Containers to hold the solutions, once made.
* Chlorine bleach.
* Clean water.
* A measuring cup.

Pour water to reach the level of the ninth mark you made on the container. Add bleach to reach the tenth mark. Simple as that; you now have 10% bleach solution.

Walls and floors can be disinfected with weaker solutions. Soap and water are reasonable items for general cleaning purposes. Remember that doorknobs, sinks, and even children's toys should be regularly disinfected. It's important to know that bleach loses strength over time, even in its original container. Expect a decrease in effectiveness after 6-12 months.

Bathroom facilities for the sick should be separate from those for the healthy, if possible. Have closed containers like hampers to put used sick room items that need to be cleaned.

A station near the entrance of the room for masks and gloves would be very useful. In the case of highly contagious diseases spread by bodily fluids, gowns, aprons, and face shields should be considered. These are commercially available but can be improvised as well.

At your entry station, you'll need a basin with water, soap, hand sanitizer, and towels for exclusive use by the caregiver. There should only be only one person involved in caring for infectious disease cases.

The sick room that is geared to deal with infections does not have to include tourniquets and gauze bandages. It does, however, have to include sheets, towels, pillows, utensils, and other items for the exclusive use of the patient. Keep these items separate from the bedding, bathing, and eating materials of the healthy members of your family.

Consider bedding and clothes of the ill to be infected, and wash your hands right after touching them or the patient. Any equipment brought into the sick room should stay there.

One additional item that will be important to your sick room patients: Give them a noisemaker of some sort that will allow them to alert you when they need help. This will decrease anxiety and give them confidence that you will know when they are in need of your presence.

Now You Know: Now you know a lot about the exclusive list of pandemic diseases that Zika virus has apparently joined. You learned about viruses, bacteria, and protozoa, and what makes an infectious disease pandemic, epidemic, or endemic. You learned the basics of how your body's immunity works.

You also learned about pandemic diseases in world history, and the methods by which they can be transmitted besides just mosquito bites. You know which diseases are likely to be candidates for the next pandemic, including a number of related mosquito-borne infections. You can now put together an effective sick room in case an epidemic affects your community.

PART 3

Preventing Zika Virus

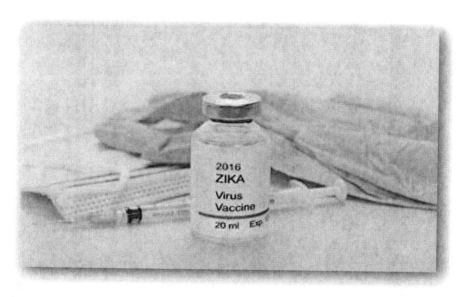

IN THE CASE OF VIRAL diseases, there are no cures and only a few drugs that will have a positive effect on the course of certain illnesses like influenza. This is especially true in the case of Zika virus. The Center for Disease Control and Prevention states simply, "There is no vaccine to prevent or specific medicine to treat Zika infections". At best, you can use acetaminophen (Tylenol) to treat fevers and muscle aches and drink fluids to stay hydrated.

This doesn't mean that nothing can be done to combat it. The president of the United States has ask congress for 1.8 billion dollars for specific programs to prepare communities at risk for a possible epidemic. Countries in Europe are also considering putting resources into research and control.

The Vaccine Vacuum

In an age where there seems to be a vaccine (and an accompanying controversy) for every pandemic disease, it is hard to believe that there isn't one available against the Zika virus. Vaccines have been developed against many of the infections that have caused serious health threats in the past. The recent recognition of the threat that ZIKV poses is a signal to medical researchers to produce an effective form of prevention.

Governments and pharmaceutical companies have taken notice and are feverishly working to move on this project. Albertina Torsoli and Rebecca Spaulding discuss these efforts in Bloomberg Business:

"...These days, the virus has sparked a gold rush of its own: companies are touting products from vaccines not even tried in mice to devices that filter Zika from the blood -- leaving public health experts to determine which proposals can help halt the mosquito-borne disease's explosive spread.

More than 15 companies have been in touch with the World Health Organization about developing vaccines, and about 20 are working on diagnostic tools..."

U.S. president Barack Obama has asked congress for money to fund research and other countries are following suit. Seeing an opportunity, the world's pharmaceutical companies are racing to put out a vaccine and new tests for ZIKV, including France's Sanofi (which developed a vaccine against Dengue Fever, a related virus), the United States' Inovio Pharmaceuticals and GeoVax

Labs, and India's Bharat Biotech. Even the National Institute of Health (NIH) has made it a priority to develop a vaccine and new testing.

Despite the efforts being made, a vaccine is still thought to be years away. As such, companies that make condoms are now marketing their products as effective ways to prevent a Zika-infected pregnancy.

Mosquito Control

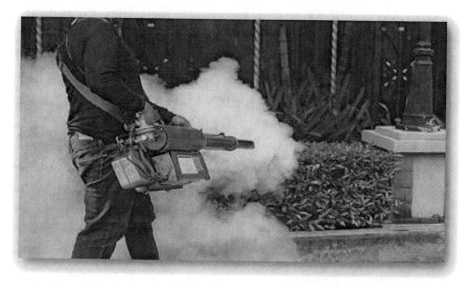

Clearly, your best strategy is prevention. As the Zika virus is caused primarily by mosquito bites, the most sensible way to prevent it is to eliminate the vector: The Aedes mosquito.

This is no easy task. The Aedes mosquito has increased its range over the last three decades to include every tropical or sub-tropical region on Earth. There is evidence that it has lately adapted itself to more temperate climates. There is even a population of Aedes mosquitoes that has survived at least four winters in Washington, D.C.

Pretty amazing for an insect whose lifespan is between two and four weeks. Some believe that they hide in underground structures like subways when the weather gets cold. This allows them to even survive blizzards and continue to reproduce.

Even if warm sanctuaries aren't available, the Aedes mosquito can survive. The mosquito itself doesn't live long enough to make it to the following spring, but its eggs can be viable for over a year. Although they are laid in water, the eggs can survive in a dry state. This gets them through winters and dry spells, with hatching occurring during the next rain.

The presence of mosquitoes is no surprise, but it's important to know when new species arrive to an area or the current residents are having a population explosion. Knowing when breeding activity is highest is also a key.

Adult mosquito populations are monitored in a number of ways. Mechanical traps using carbon dioxide or lactic acid, compounds emitted by humans, are helpful for collection purposes. An older method simply uses a human subject who counts the number of times that a mosquito lands on their arms or legs in a certain time interval.

Monitoring larval (juvenile) mosquito populations involves collecting larvae from standing water. The total number of larvae, pupae, and species are noted for each collection. An alternative method of collection involves putting out pots of standing water with black cardboard that serve as artificial egg-laying platforms. These are sometimes called "ovitraps"; they "trap" the eggs in a container that can be removed from the area for study.

Once the threat of mosquito-borne disease is identified in an area, a decision must be made as to how to control the population. Mosquito control may concentrate on eliminating adult mosquitoes, their larvae, or (preferably) both.

There are several methods of controlling mosquitoes. Usually, using a combination of methods will be most effective. Natural methods are preferable to pesticides, due to concerns about health risks to humans and the local ecology. Efforts to eliminate larvae is generally thought to be superior to killing adults.

SOURCE REDUCTION

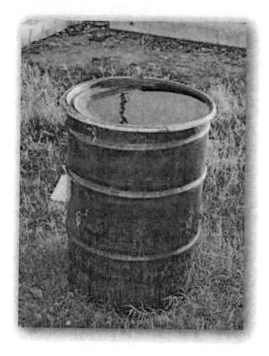

A method that eliminates both adults and larvae is called "source reduction". Source reduction is a type of environmental management that involves removing breeding habitat.

Mosquitoes breed in any collection of standing water. Lakes, swamps, and other wetlands are favorite spots. They aren't choosy, however, and will breed in ground water from a recent storm, a bucket left out in the rain, or the inside of an old tire in a junkyard. As little as one teaspoon of water (just enough to fill a bottle cap) that stands for two weeks will work just fine for the female Aedes mosquito. It takes less than 2 weeks for the larvae to become an adult.

If you're traveling to countries where Zika or other mosquito-borne outbreaks are occurring, mosquito control may mean simply staying inside buildings with air conditioning or, if you must be outside, in patios or other screened areas.

If ZIKV has been identified in your home town, you will have to take more aggressive measures. You can decrease the chance that mosquitoes will want to breed in your backyard by eliminating standing water. Consider:

* Covering rain barrels with a screen or other barrier.
* Keeping lids on garbage cans.
* Strictly maintaining disinfection in swimming pools or hot tubs using chlorine or salt. Assure that water is circulating well. Drain completely if not in use. Abandoned swimming pools should be filled in with dirt or sand.
* Emptying kiddie wading pools.

* Draining water from tarps, pool covers, or other protective sheeting.
* Removing buckets, empty flower pots, and other containers that might accumulate water.
* Frequently changing water in birdbaths, pet dishes, and animal troughs.
* Unclogging rain gutters that might not be draining well.
* Repairing any leaky outdoor faucets.
* Installing or repairing tightly-fitting window and door screens. Use U.S. #16 or #18 mesh.
* Adding a water feature to a standing pond, such as a waterfall or fountain.
* Removing debris from ornamental ponds or fountains that might prevent water flow.
* Installing or repairing tightly-fitting window and door screens.
* Cutting or mowing areas of tall grass, a favorite place for adult mosquitoes to loiter.
* Avoiding excessive watering of lawns and plants, especially near the house.
* Adding topsoil to uneven areas of your yard that might accumulate rain water.
* Notifying local authorities of nearby properties with areas of undrained storm water that could be an issue. They will probably have equipment that can eliminate the problem.

Note that draining wetlands and natural ponds may be illegal. There are many natural predators of mosquitoes that live there, such as birds, bats, fish, frogs, and other wildlife. Check with your local municipalities for rules and regulations.

BioControl

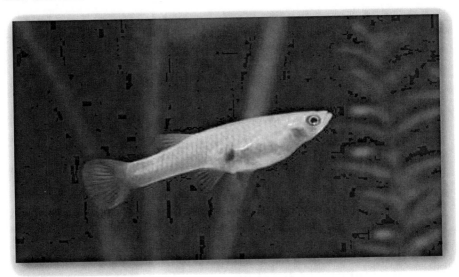

Biological control of mosquito populations involves the use of natural predators, parasites, and pathogens (disease-causing organisms). Introduction of other animals or microbes must be managed carefully to reduce negative effects on the environment.

Effective biocontrol agents include certain guppy-sized fish that include mosquito larvae in their diet. *Gambusia Affinis* (see image, also known as the "mosquitofish), tilapia, goldfish, killifish, and certain minnows are efficient curbs on the mosquito population. Be aware that adding these fish to areas where they aren't found naturally may have harmful effects on the ecology and must be employed with great caution.

Insect predators are also voracious devourers of both adult and larval mosquitoes. The juvenile dragonfly, also called a "naiad", consumes mosquito larvae while the adult dragonfly eats the adults. One mosquito species, *Toxorhynchies*, eats other mosquitoes but has had less success in thinning the population than the dragonfly.

A number of small lizards, such as the gecko, also eat adult mosquitoes. Frogs and other amphibians are also an option. Fresh water crustaceans such as crayfish may also be a welcome addition to eat larvae, but their effectiveness in control is not yet proven.

Certain small birds, such as swallows, include adult mosquitoes in their diet, and bats also consider them a food item. Few studies, however, have been performed to determine how well they would perform as a biocontrol agent.

Although mosquitoes don't feel any ill effects from carrying Zika virus, they are vulnerable to disease like any other creature. Bacteria, protozoa, viruses, nematodes, and fungi cause damage to mosquito populations.

One biological method that has been shown to be effective for large-scale mosquito control is a bacteria found in the soil called *Bacillus thuringiensis israelensis* (BTI). It acts as a "larvicide" or "larvacide": An agent that kills juvenile mosquitoes. Microbial larvicides like BTI are bacteria that are registered as pesticides for control of mosquito larvae.

Added to water, BTI kills larvae by damaging their digestive system. BTI Toxins rupture cells and rapidly lead to a fatal loss of body fluids. This action occurs so quickly as to decimate larval populations in 24 hours.

It should be noted that, once larvae turn in pupae, they stop eating. BTI then becomes ineffective as a biocontrol agent. Despite this, success has been achieved with large-scale usage of BTI by dropping it in water sources by helicopter.

Bacillus sphaericus is a spore-forming bacterium found throughout the world in soil and aquatic environments. Although the method of action is similar to BTI, this bacteria works a little slower but has a more long-lasting effect.

Fungi of two species, *Metarhizium anisopliae* and *Beauveria bassiana* are known to kill adult mosquitoes. They act as parasites to infect, not only mosquitoes, but termites, whiteflies, and other harmful insects.

Biological control of mosquitoes can be achieved by introducing another animal into their habitat: its own species. Males sterilized with radiation or other methods are released into the environment and mate with females without producing any young. This has worked well in various programs.

The latest technology involves modifying the genetic material of the mosquito to decrease its population or success in its range. Oxford University, through its subsidiary Oxitec, has genetically modified the *Aedes Aegypti* male mosquito. It introduced a gene into lab-bred male mosquitoes that causes any offspring to die before reaching adulthood. This modified male (known as OX513A) is released into the environment in quantity to compete with other males for mating privileges.

What would be the effect of one Aedes female mating with an OX513A male? One female could, over its month-long life span, produce 500 offspring. If all the offspring survived, the next generation could number 125,000, and the next in the millions.

Genetically-modified mosquitoes have been used in the Florida Keys to combat mosquito populations with some success, and is now being employed in Brazil and other countries in the ZIKV outbreak zone. Some areas claim more than 90% success in reducing the numbers of mosquitoes.

It should be noted that there are still environmental concerns regarding introduction of genetically modified organisms (GMOs) into an area. An important consideration, however, is that the *Aedes Aegypti* and *Aedes Albopictus* species are not naturally-occurring inhabitants of the Western Hemisphere. That means they aren't meant to be part of the ecology there. More research is needed to determine the effect of GMO insects and to weigh risks and benefits of their use.

CHEMICAL CONTROL OF LARVAE

Chemical pesticides are a time-honored way to reduce mosquito populations.

Mosquito larvicides registered for use in Florida are discussed below within the following classification system:

* Insect growth regulators (IGRs)
* Organophosphates (OPs)
* Surface oils and films

Insect growth regulators: a natural juvenile hormone (JH) that allows normal metamorphosis from the larval to the adult insect was discovered in 1967. This hormone doesn't exist in higher animals, so a chemical that had an effect on JH was considered a possibly effective pesticide. One such chemical (Methoprene) was found that appeared to block the ability of the larval mosquito to develop into the adult. As well, it appear to interfere with larval growth patterns and cause malformations.

Methoprene is absorbed through the insect's "skin" or may be incidentally ingested. When Methoprene was added to the water habitat in a higher level than the juvenile hormone in the larva's body, pupae were not able to emerge as adults and, since they don't eat, eventually starved to death.

ORGANOPHOSPHATES

The word "organophosphate" (OP) refers to any pesticide containing phosphorus. OPs were first discovered during a search for a substitute for nicotine, which was once used as an insecticide around World War II. Organophosphates have been used for mosquito and other insect control since the early 1950s.

OPs enter the body of a target organisms and damage nerve cells in the insect. The organophosphate causes a loss of coordination which progresses to paralysis and eventual death.

Temephos is an OP compound. During the 1960s, it was studied as a replacement for the controversial insecticide DDT in malaria control programs. Temephos was often recommended to use in rotation with Methoprene in integrated pest management efforts. It was considered one of the few organophosphates effective against Aedes mosquito larvae. Unfortunately, recent studies suggest that some larval populations may be exhibiting resistance to the substance. It's unfortunate because most believe that Temephos, one of the few OPs available as a larvacide, was one of the few organophosphates that has little or no detrimental effects on non-target organisms like mammals; some health organizations even believe that it is safe when used in drinking water.

Temephos use is being discontinued in the U.S., but it is still in use in other countries. Although it may not be sold by the manufacturer anymore, existing stocks may be utilized until exhausted.

SURFACE OILS AND FILMS

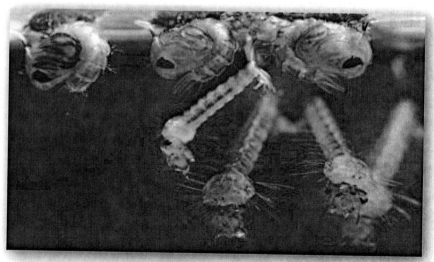

Both the larva and pupa of mosquitoes must breathe air from the surface

One of the first larvicides ever used, surface oils and films such as diesel, kerosene, and motor oil have been around since the 1930s. Since that time, newer thin layer surface films and highly refined oils have been developed that are virtually colorless and odorless. They are also much thinner than older oils and films without losing effectiveness against mosquito larvae.

Surface oils and films are meant to suffocate larvae as they come up for air. One gallon is sufficient to treat an acre and provides control over the course of a week. Larger quantities seem to accelerate the process. Surface oils are considered a satisfactory method for pupal control and can eliminate newly emerged adults on the water's surface.

There are disadvantages to using some of these products. Effectiveness is limited to those species which breathe air at the water surface. A visible oil slick is noticeable on the water and some have an objectionable odor and appearance. As such, they are not used in waters used for human consumption.

The newest surface films are called Monomolecular films (MMFs). These are alcohol-based and biodegradable products made from renewable plant oils. MMFs produce an extremely thin film on the water's surface. When applied, they quickly spread over the surface of the water to form a film about one molecule in thickness. They are colorless and odorless.

MMFs act by significantly reducing the surface tension of the water and drowning mosquito larvae and adults. The film causes difficulty with proper positioning at the water-air border, which causes multiple issues: larvae, pupae, emerging adults, and female landing on the surface to lay eggs drown; eggs can't float normally, sink to the bottom, and don't hatch.

Monomolecular firms don't appear to affect fish and other wildlife. They remain active for up to 2 weeks in standing water.

New Technology

After generations of using chemical pesticides, a new method of killing mosquito larvae known as an "acoustic larvicide" is being developed.

Acoustic larvicides use a technique where sound waves are used at certain frequencies in larval mosquito habitats. The air bladders in the larvae burst, killing them, when exposed to the sound at these frequency levels. Further study is required to determine the effects of acoustic larvicides on species other than mosquitoes.

Further use of genetic modification may play a role in the control of mosquito larva populations. Research is under way to modify genes in certain aquatic plants so that they emit a larvacide. Concerns include the effect on water quality and the effect on non-target inhabitants of wetlands.

One last strategy involves inserting a gene that makes mosquito eggs glow when exposed to ultraviolet light, making them easier to identify.

ADULT MOSQUITO CONTROL

The Zika virus epidemic has reached the point that many affected countries are mounting concerted efforts to eliminate the Aedes mosquito population. Beside source reduction (discussed earlier) to reduce breeding habitat, destroying the existing adult mosquito population has become a main goal.

Biocontrol in the form of genetically-modified adult male mosquitoes is seeing some success in eliminating large numbers. Chemical pesticides, however, are still being used in many areas for an immediate effect on the adult mosquito population. These include organophosphates and pyrethroids.

Although expensive in terms of manpower, equipment, and inventory, large scale spraying with "adulticides" is the main method that quickly reduces mosquito numbers or reaches otherwise inaccessible breeding areas.

ORGANOPHOSPHATE SPRAYS

Malathion: Malathion 5% is an "adulticide"; that is, it kills adult mosquitoes once they have emerged from the pupal stage. It is applied in large-scale mosquito control programs from sprayers mounted on trucks and aircraft. To decrease the effect on the environment, Malathion is used as an ultra-low volume (ULV) spray. ULV sprayers release very fine aerosol droplets that stay in the air and kill mosquitoes on contact. Less than 4 ounces of Malathion is required to cover an acre of land.

Because of the very small amount of active ingredient released, there are few circumstances in which Malathion would cause damage to humans or animals. Exposure to high amounts of organophosphate, however, can cause irritation to the nervous system. Symptoms include nausea and dizziness. Exposure to extremely high quantities can cause seizures and be life-threatening. Luckily, Malathion degrades rapidly once it reaches the ground.

Naled: Naled is another organophosphate (OP) used primarily for controlling adult mosquitoes, Like Malathion, Naled is applied by truck or aircraft-mounted ULV sprayers. Only 0.1 pound of active ingredient is required per acre of land to be fumigated. Naled is at least as safe as Malathion when used in appropriate quantities.

PYRETHROIDS

Pyrethroids are synthetic insecticide versions of pyrethrins, a natural compound derived from chrysanthemum flowers that is sometimes used in the control of human lice. Some commonly used pyrethroids in mosquito control programs are permethrin, resmethrin, and d-phenothrin (Sumithrin).

Permethrin: Permethrin is sold in a number of products such as indoor and outdoor insect foggers and sprays that kill on contact. A number of different insects are repelled by clothing treated with this substance, but it is to be avoided on the skin except for specific circumstances. Permethrin is the most widely used mosquito adulticide in the United States, due to its low cost and high success rate.

In fact, 10 million acres of U.S. land are sprayed with permethrin every year.

Resmethrin: Resmethrin is registered for use in public health and vector control programs to control adult mosquitos and some biting flies. Because of its toxicity to fish, resmethrin is no longer available for use after January 1, 2016, except for products already purchased.

D-phenothrin: D-phenothrin (Sumithrin) has been in use to control adult mosquitos and other nuisance insects indoors and in outdoor public and private areas. It has been widely used around residential buildings and has been used for direct treatment on dogs.

It should be noted that, in addition to some pyrethroids being toxic to fish, damage to pollinator bee populations have also occurred after spraying. Use of chemical sprays should only be undertaken with consideration given to the environment.

The use of long-lasting chemical sprays on both outside and inside walls of buildings acts to kill adult mosquitoes as they land on these structures to rest. They are also applied to roofs. Indoor foggers have been used with success in problem areas. The interior compartments of commercial aircraft have also been the target of some indoor spraying efforts.

Any discussion of chemical pesticides should include a mention of one of the first ones developed in the 19th century: **DDT**. An organochlorine, DDT lethally damaged the nervous system of insects. It was used to prevent malaria outbreaks in allied troops during World

War II. After the war, it found use in agriculture and became the primary chemical insecticide for decades.

Over time, the environmental impact of DDT revealed significant ill effects on wildlife, especially birds, and even a link to cancer in humans. Public outcry led to the beginnings of the environmentalist movement and the passage of the Endangered Species Act. In 1972, DDT was banned from use in the United States.

Since then, DDT has been banned globally except for some underdeveloped countries where it is still used in mosquito control programs.

Mosquito Traps

Non-chemical methods of trapping mosquitoes may be an option for small properties or the private home. A number of mechanical traps are commercially available, some of which use propane to generate carbon dioxide and heat to attract the adult female mosquito. Some carbon dioxide traps even produce similar quantities seen in human exhalation.

These attractants lure the mosquito into the "trap", which is often a net or an adhesive board on which the mosquito becomes stuck. Sometimes, a vacuum fan sucks the mosquito into the trap, where they dehydrate and die.

Carbon dioxide traps are promising as they attract insects that feed on blood from human hosts. It's important to note, however, that carbon dioxide traps shouldn't be placed near where humans will be, as the mosquito will be lured directly to its hosts and may prefer them instead.

Other traps are "zappers" that kill insects with an electric shock. These are inferior in that they are indiscriminate with regards to the species of insect killed. In addition, the attractant in electronic bug killers is light, something to which mosquitoes are not particularly attracted.

In one study, 14,000 insects were "zapped", but when evaluated to determine what insects were killed, only 30 of them were mosquitoes. Another showed that, of the insects killed by these devices, only 0.13% were female mosquitoes (males don't bite humans). An estimated 70-350 billion insects, many beneficial, are killed annually in the United States by these electrocuting devices.

Mechanical traps like the ones described require some level of maintenance and need to be emptied and cleaned. Some components like adhesive boards must be replaced regularly for the trap to maintain its effectiveness.

In view of the costs involved in the purchase of some mechanical traps, a number of homemade traps have been proposed. These use fermented fruit juice as bait and are engineered to allow mosquitoes and other insects in, but not out. While they certainly trap a lot of insects, they are as likely to attract bees and fruit flies as mosquitoes.

MISTING SYSTEMS

Outdoor misting systems are designed to spray pesticides in a fine mist to kill mosquitoes and other insects. They are usually reserved for homes and businesses. Misting systems use nozzles mounted around a perimeter of a property and connected by tubing to a reservoir of pesticide, usually a pyrethroid. Many spray at preset intervals.

Misting systems are considered to be the ultimate in high-tech mosquito control, but there are significant concerns. The American Mosquito Control Association (AMCA) believes that it is important to note the limitations and risks of misting systems. Here are their concerns:

- **Unnecessary insecticide use.** Users of these systems don't have the resources to monitor the number and density of local mosquito species. Thus, timed space sprays may result in needless insecticide applications, which leads to increased costs to the consumer and possibly negative environmental impacts.
- **Lack of efficacy data.** There is little data to demonstrate that misting systems actually serve to control mosquito populations even when using insecticides.
- **Non-target impacts.** Timed-release sprays will negatively impact beneficial insect populations on site and through uncontrolled off-site drift.
- **Promotion of insecticide resistance.** The indiscriminate application of pyrethrins will likely lead to the development of resistance on the part of mosquitoes, which have been known

to mutate. Since pyrethroids play an essential role as a mosquito adulticide, resistance to these compounds may have dire consequences for the control of mosquito-borne illnesses like Zika virus.

* **Risk of pesticide exposure.** Most misting systems lack safeguards to prevent inhalation and other exposures to children, pets, and wildlife. Even though a disclaimer may exist on the system's label, mishaps due to negligence can occur.

The AMCA also notes that misting systems are incompatible with good integrated pest management practices. The hands-off nature of these products will tempt homeowners to avoid important source reduction methods of reducing the mosquito populations, like draining standing water or using personal insect repellants.

COMMUNITY EFFORTS

Mosquito issues that affect the general population often cannot be eliminated through the efforts of individual homeowners. Therefore many local, county, and state authorities have in place some form of organized mosquito control. There are approximately 734 organized mosquito control organizations in the United States. In addition, more than a thousand residential communities have programs dedicated to controlling mosquito problems.

There has been an increase in the urgency on the part of municipalities in the last twenty years to achieve mosquito control, corresponding to the first West Nile virus outbreak in 1999. These organized management programs incorporate the integrated pest management strategies mentioned in this book.

Permanent measures include large-scale operations such as draining swamps and other mosquito breeding areas. Efforts concentrate on killing larvae with larvicides and aerosol spraying by ground or aerial equipment to kill adults.

Municipalities can't act, however, if they aren't aware of the problem. If you live in an area with a large mosquito population, you must encourage a public effort. Organized mosquito management can accomplish much more than anything you can do on your own. Contact local health officials to initiate action against mosquito-borne disease.

Some feel that, if a significant outbreak occurs in the U.S., it may be more difficult to control that in Brazil. In South America, many programs go into individual homes and spray the walls with pesticide. This would meet significant public resistance in the United States, however, and may even be illegal in some areas.

Protecting the Pregnant Woman

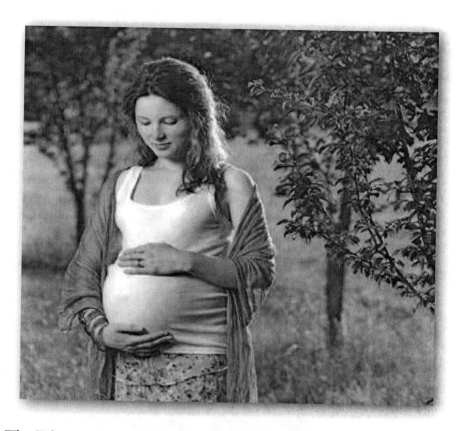

The Zika virus causes a relatively minor illness, except when a pregnant woman is exposed at the stage when the fetus is undergoing major brain development. Although not completely proven, the number of newborns in ZIKV epidemic zones with microcephaly may be indicative of a connection with the virus.

It's important to protect everyone from the projected millions of case of Zika virus disease, but it's especially important to protect those that are expecting. Specific strategies must be developed to decrease the risk of microcephaly as much as humanly possible.

For those pregnant women in the United States or other countries where there is not a large number of local transmission of the disease, the most effective way of preventing Zika is simple: Stay home.

Almost all Zika cases diagnosed in American citizens have been in those who recently returned from trips to affected countries like Brazil. As a result, the United States has issued a travel advisory to pregnant women to postpone travel to any country with an outbreak.

This should probably, as a precaution, also pertain to women who are considering pregnancy. At the very least, the subject should be discussed with their healthcare provider.

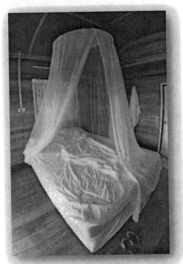

Mosquito netting

If you must travel to countries where Zika virus outbreaks are occurring, take the following steps:

* Wear long-sleeved shirts and long pants.
* Stay in places with air conditioning or, at least, window and door screening.
* Sleep under a mosquito net if you must be outside.
* Even though Aedes mosquitoes can bite any time of the day, stay indoors during the peak mosquito hours at dawn and dusk. Aedes mosquitoes generally feed less often at night.

Given the World Health Organization's prediction of 4 million cases of ZIKV with possible 100,000 newborns afflicted, it stands to reason that some of these cases might originate in the United States. Certainly, the *Aedes Aegypti* and *Aedes Albopictus* mosquitoes that transmit the virus have a strong foothold in many areas of the country. This raises the possibility that Zika virus disease outbreaks might occur in U.S. communities.

In that circumstance, staying home isn't a sure way to prevent becoming infected. The pregnant woman must take additional steps to prevent being bitten by a mosquito with the virus.

The American Mosquito Control Association suggests the three D's: **Drain, Dress, and Defend**. We discussed the first D, "Drain", in our section on source reduction, and that protects the home. We must now consider personal strategies to prevent becoming the next victim of the Zika virus.

The second D is for "Dress". Mosquitoes are attracted to the heat absorbed by very dark clothing, so it makes sense to wear light colors.

Some mosquitoes can bite right through tight-fitting clothes, so your ensemble should fit loosely. Woven fabrics like nylon or polyester seems to provide more protection than knit fabrics.

Most important, perhaps, is to wear long sleeves and pants. Avoid exposing as much skin as possible if a mosquito-borne illness has invaded your town. Tuck shirts into pants, and pants into socks; this will fully cover any open gaps in clothing.

Another option is to treat your clothing with a pesticide called permethrin. The U.S. Military has used permethrin-treated clothing for decades to protect soldiers in epidemic zones.

When applied properly to clothes, permethrin binds tightly to fabrics. So tightly, in fact, that it withstands laundering with minimal transfer to skin.

Here are some tips when using permethrin to treat clothing for mosquito protection:

- Read instructions carefully and don't use more of the product that the directions recommend.
- Make certain that the permethrin product you use has specific instructions for treating clothing. Every permethrin product may not do for clothing.
- Don't use permethrin on clothing while it's being worn.
- Don't apply the product indoors. Only use outside in areas protected from wind.
- Hang your treated clothing outdoors after spraying and don't wear them until they are completely dry.

✴ Wash all your permethrin-treated clothes separate from other items.

Another item you could wear to prevent mosquito bites are "mosquito bracelets" and other commercially available items. Some can be worn on belt loops or waistbands. These reportedly contain repellants or other substances that decrease your risk of bites. Unfortunately, there is a lack of evidence of any efficacy in preventing bites in any area with large numbers of mosquitoes.

Now, you're dressed for success against mosquito bites. This leads us to our last D, for "Defend". Exposed skin must be defended with mosquito repellant.

Mosquito Repellants

Mosquito repellant is meant to repel mosquitoes, but doesn't kill them. Used correctly, repellants are very effective in preventing bites, even when there are large quantities of mosquitoes nearby.

It's best to choose a product registered by the Environmental Protection Agency (EPA). These are approved for human use and must pass rigorous safety guidelines. Most importantly for the purposes of this book, they are safe for pregnant and breastfeeding women. The repellants recommended by the EPA are:

✴ DEET (N, N-diethyl-meta-toluamide)
✴ Picaridin (KBR 3023)

* IR3535 (Ethyl butylacetylaminopropionate)
* Oil of lemon eucalyptus (p-methane 3,8-diol)

DEET: For some reason, both male and female mosquitoes intensely dislike the smell of DEET. It appears to confuse them and they are unable to land on human hosts.

Consumer Reports magazine found a direct correlation between the concentration of DEET used and the numbers of hours of protection against insect bites. 20-34% DEET gave from 3-6 hours of protection; 100% DEET, on the other hand, gave up to 24 hours of protection. Some people note skin irritation from DEET, especially if it is used under clothes.

The CDC states that sunscreen and DEET repellant can, and should, be used at the same time, especially in warm areas where Zika has been documented. Apply sunscreen first, then DEET. The CDC recommends using individual products as opposed to DEET and sunscreen combinations.

The Centers for Disease Control and Prevention recommends 30-50% formulations to prevent the spread of mosquito-borne diseases like ZIKV.

Picaridin: Also called Icaridin, was synthesized to resemble the natural compound piperine, which is found in black pepper. Picaridin appears to block mosquitoes from sensing humans and makes them less likely to bite. Some preparations of Picaridin are not as long-lasting as DEET, and more frequent reapplication may be needed.

IR3535: A synthetic compound that is also classified as a biopesticide by the Environmental Protection Agency.

Lemon Eucalyptus Oil: Oil from the lemon eucalyptus tree is effective against mosquito bites and even provides protection against the deer tick, which carries the Lyme disease microbe.

A 2006 Consumer Reports article compared lemon eucalyptus oil favorably to low concentration DEET products. Each application gives about two hours of protection.

Here are some basic tips when using mosquito repellants:

* Read the directions before applying.
* Apply repellent lightly on exposed skin (not on clothing).
* Keep repellents away from eyes, lips, and nostrils.
* Don't inhale or ingest repellents.
* Avoid using repellents on wounds or irritated skin.
* Repeat light applications of repellant as needed throughout the day.
* Wash skin after coming indoors.
* Call your physician if you notice a reaction on repellant-treated skin.

For children:

* Use 30% DEET or lower on young children. DEET can be used on infants 2 months of age or older.

* Don't apply repellants to palms of hands, which are likely to have contact with the mouth or eyes.
* Spray repellant on your hands and use them to apply on the child's face. If an infant, cover baby strollers with netting for additional protection.

NATURAL MOSQUITO REPELLANTS

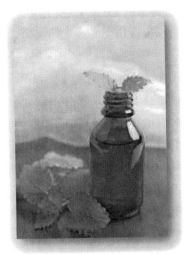

Although lemon eucalyptus oil is the only natural product officially recommended by the EPA as a mosquito repellant, a number of other substances found in nature have also been documented to have a similar effect:

CITRONELLA

A well-known natural mosquito repellent. Oil of citronella is the most common ingredient used in mosquito repellant candles and incense you'll find in home stores. By itself, the candles decrease mosquito bites by 40%, but the plant is also used to make lotions and sprays which should be used in addition for higher level of protection.

Leaves from citronella plants can be rubbed on the skin for protection, although a small percentage of people may notice mild irritation.

GERANIUM

The *New England Journal of Medicine* study found that a repellent containing geranium oil was as effective as low concentration DEET products.

CLOVE

In a 2005 study that compared the repellent activity of 38 different essential oils, researchers discovered that products containing clove oil offered the longest duration of protection against all mosquito species involved in the lab experiments. It should be noted that pure clove oil should not be applied to skin, as it may have adverse effects.

Other natural products being investigated for their ability to repel insects include:

* Fennel
* Thyme
* Rosemary
* Garlic

* Neem
* Celery extract

If you're considering the use of any natural mosquito remedy, talk to your doctor first to discuss your options.

Obstetric Care

Good prenatal care of pregnant women in zones that are experiencing Zika outbreaks is one of the keys to identifying the acute disease and its serious effects on the fetus. There is no evidence that pregnant women are more likely to get ZIKV than men or non-pregnant women. Despite this, some believe that pregnant women exhale more carbon dioxide, a powerful attractant to mosquitoes.

The CDC has updated its guidelines for healthcare providers caring for pregnant women and women that might become pregnant during outbreaks of Zika virus. These guidelines apply to healthcare providers not only for the United States, but its territories as well. These guidelines are fluid and will likely change as we learn more about ZIKV.

A new recommendation by the CDC for obstetricians and midwives is to offer blood tests to pregnant women who do not report symptoms of illness consistent with Zika virus disease. Testing should be considered in all pregnant women who have traveled to areas where Zika is being reported. This is because 80% of women will not have symptoms of the acute illness, which presents as fever, headache, joint pain, and conjunctivitis ("pink eye").

The guidelines state that testing should be offered between 2 and 12 weeks after pregnant women return to the U.S. The updated guidelines also include suggestions for screening, testing, and care of pregnant women, as well as recommendations for counseling women of reproductive age, defined as 15-44 years of age.

IgM antibody testing for Zika virus, previously mentioned in this book, is helpful to identify previous exposure. Data from previous studies of related viruses suggest that this testing may be useful when the time of exposure is known.

A negative IgM test result 2-12 weeks after known exposure suggests that a recent Zika virus infection did not occur. A positive test could still mean a different virus in the same family, like Dengue fever, is the cause. Further testing will identify Zika specifically. These results will help local health officials determine the time and frequency of ultrasound exams to identify possible Zika effects on the fetus, such as microcephaly.

If a pregnant woman has symptoms of ZiKV currently, a blood test known as reverse transcriptase-polymerase chain reaction (RT-PCR) must be performed. This test is not yet available locally in most areas of the U.S., and should be arranged with the CDC or one of several state labs that are equipped to run the study. Suspected ZIKV cases must be reported to local health officials, who can help arrange needed tests. Testing can go beyond just examining the blood. The placenta can be examined after delivery of the baby.

Zika virus can be transmitted from a pregnant mother to her fetus during pregnancy or around the time of delivery (the "perinatal" period). It is not known how often Zika perinatal transmission occurs or how often Zika is passed sexually during pregnancy. The risk for sexual transmission of Zika virus can be eliminated by abstinence and reduced by the use of condoms. This practice is officially recommended by the CDC for any male who has traveled to the Zika zone and has a pregnant partner.

As Zika virus is also associated with a syndrome called Guillain-Barre, pregnant women should report muscle weakness, numbness, and other nerve-related symptoms. Guillain-Barre, mentioned earlier, is an autoimmune condition where the body attacks its own nervous system. The exact reason why Guillain-Barre syndrome sometimes occurs with ZIKV is not yet known.

Practitioners who care for pregnant women should encourage the use of EPA-recommended mosquito repellants to avoid bites. These repellants are not only safe for pregnant women, but are also a reasonable recommendation to partners who may pass Zika sexually to the patient.

In these days of new mosquito-borne viruses, caregivers should discuss appropriate mosquito control methods as well as encourage coverage with long sleeves and pants. Medical professionals should also learn basic ways to decrease exposure to mosquitoes using source reduction as discussed earlier.

The CDC recommends that pregnant women in any trimester should consider postponing travel to an area where Zika virus transmission is ongoing. Obstetric care providers should be notified if a pregnant women is considering travel to epidemic zones. If she travels, she should strictly follow steps to avoid mosquito bites during the trip and arrange for testing soon after arriving home.

The main concern for healthcare providers is the possibility of a baby born with microcephaly. Although evidence of a relationship between Zika virus and this birth defect exists, it has not yet been proven beyond a shadow of a doubt. Research is ongoing. No other negative pregnancy outcome has been identified so far.

The most non-invasive method of evaluating a baby is serial ultrasounds. Fetal ultrasound is a routine part of prenatal care and is usually performed around 18-20 weeks. Measurements of head circumference are performed that will indicate abnormalities in growth. Ultrasound can also identify the presence of calcifications in the eyes or head, another sign of possible infection.

Several ultrasound exams throughout the pregnancy will allow the identification of continuing head growth or the lack of it, or the development of calcifications. Microcephaly is best confirmed by measuring the growth progress of the fetal head over time. There is no evidence that there is any ill effect to mother or baby as a result of ultrasound testing, even if done serially.

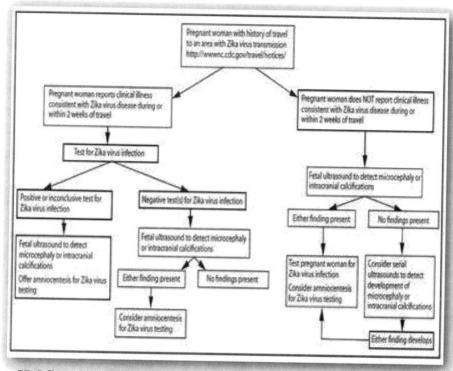

CDC flow chart for diagnosis of Zika in women returning from affected areas

Although Zika is possibly associated with the abnormality, microcephaly can be caused by other factors, including genetic issues. Amniocentesis can identify many of these. Amniocentesis is a procedure where fluid from inside the uterus is obtained and sent for testing. It identifies genetic problems like Down's syndrome as well as the presence of infections.

From a Zika standpoint, the procedure should be offered to pregnant women who experienced symptoms of acute illness during their travels or have evidence of microcephaly on ultrasound exam. Amniocentesis is safest when performed after the 15th week of pregnancy.

If the United States starts seeing outbreaks of locally-transmitted infections, all pregnant women in the community should be tested, especially those with symptoms. This should be performed at the first prenatal visit and then again in the middle of the second trimester (4-6 months) or once symptoms appear. Although universal testing will tax the resources of the few labs able to perform testing, more facilities will become equipped to handle the volume if it becomes clear that there will be an increased need.

PART 4

Theories and Policies

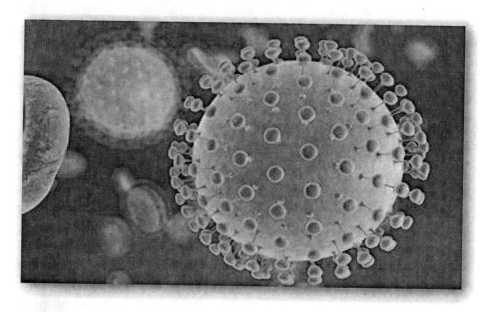

HUMANS HAVE A NATURAL TENDENCY to be inquisitive, and our efforts to understand disease have led to major progress on many medical fronts. We are just now learning about Zika virus and its newly-designated title of "pandemic".

Why should this virus, previously a minor nuisance, suddenly have changed to become capable of causing devastating effects on so many families in the New World? We hear a lot of reports of "what" and "where", but not a lot about "why". It's time to ask why.

Did Zika Mutate?

Much of the news related to the Zika virus in Brazil and other Western Hemisphere countries pertains to its possible potential to cause the birth defect microcephaly. Studies of stillborn fetuses with the abnormality have shown the present of the virus in some, and a causal link has been suggested (but not proven).

Zika virus does not originate in South America, but in Africa and Asia, where two different strains appear to exist. The Asian version is the likely strain that has crossed the Atlantic and caused cases here.

Interestingly, in Africa, Asia, and French Polynesia, Zika virus is thought to be a mild pest, causing minor illness; in fact, 80% of those infected have no symptoms at all. It is not associated with a large number of birth defects like microcephaly where it is tradition-ally found. Only now have cases of microcephaly and other brain abnormalities been found, in hindsight, in some Pacific islands.

Zika *has* been shown to occasionally cause a rare nerve disorder called "Guillain-Barre Syndrome", which presents with muscle weak-ness leading to possible paralysis. Some recover fully, but many have long-term issues and 5% die from respiratory arrest and other com-plications. Guillain-Barre is not, by the way, a disease ordinarily as-sociated with pregnancy.

Yet, this virus is now becoming an issue that the World Health Organization predicts may lead to millions of cases of acute illness and affect up to 100,000 newborns. It isn't hard to imagine that this will tax the resources of poor countries that are dealing with it.

The question that very few has asked is, "Why is a virus that isn't a big problem in its original territory suddenly causing these heartbreaking deformities?" Zika is an equatorial disease spread by Aedes mosquitoes. The climate conditions that are favorable for this mosquito are present in Brazil, Asia, and Africa. Why should ZIKV have so different a presentation in one part of the world than another?

Is it possible that we dealing with a viral "mutation"? Viruses are well-known for their ability to change genetically. These changes are called mutations and may either be insignificant or have major consequences. Luckily, most viral mutations have little effect on how contagious it is or how deadly.

The human immune system uses a number of tactics to fight viruses. The virus wants to circumvent the immune system, create copies of itself, and then spread to other hosts. Things that help a virus accomplish its goals tend to be kept from one generation to another, and may mutate to become even more efficient.

Some mutations might be too efficient. If a virus mutates in such a fashion that it kills the host very quickly, the host might not be able to infect others before it dies. In these cases, the characteristics of the new mutation will be unlikely to survive in new generations.

The concept of mutation is important to consider when it comes to viral illnesses. The basis of most vaccines is based on the theory that there is little change in a virus from one year to the next. This is the reason why influenza vaccines work to prevent illness.

This year's flu is usually similar to last year's, and flu vaccines are made from components of last year's virus. Inoculation with such a vaccine will give immunity (usually 60-70% of the time) the next time a flu virus arrives in your community.

When viruses mutate little and are relatively similar from year to year, it is called **antigenic drift**. In these cases, most of those who become very ill are the elderly or, sometimes, the very young. Healthy young specimens are able to fight off the virus easily.

When a major mutation occurs, we call it **antigenic shift.** These mutations change the virus in a significant manner, and we see it affect healthy young adults seriously more often. When an antigenic shift occurs, viruses become killers or cause entirely different effects.

For example, a virus that was previously only transmissible through body fluids may become airborne. A virus that causes a mild flu-like syndrome could cause severe pneumonias instead. Because we haven't developed resistance to the new version's reproduction in the body, society is presented with a major threat.

In cases of antigenic shift, vaccines become less effective. The virus causes more severe outbreaks that medical facilities are sometimes hard pressed to manage. Indeed, these mutations are often the cause of killer pandemics.

Imagine if Ebola, which caused a regional epidemic in West Africa in 2014, had mutated to become easily transmissible through the air? It would have been more challenging to control and could have reached pandemic status. Indeed, a number of mutations were noted in the Ebola virus, but fortunately, they didn't change the disease significantly or the effectiveness of treatments or newly developed vaccines.

Which brings us back to Zika virus. Is it possible that the Zika virus has mutated in such a way that it now affects fetal brain development? If so, why did the mutation occur? Is there some benefit to the virus for having done so? It's difficult to see any real reason for such a mutation to occur. Mutations may occur randomly, however, without serving any real purpose. Perhaps this is exactly what happened in the case of Zika.

It's puzzling that so little thought has been given to the possibility that the virus, or the Aedes mosquito that carries it, might have mutated. Considering that it may now be causing complications with the fetus during pregnancy, you would think that this common viral characteristic would be a likely cause. It's routinely investigated in other viral outbreaks, why not Zika?

At the time of this writing, only the author's own writings pose this theory when searched online. In conferences calls with state medical authorities, however, officials cannot discount the possibility of a mutation when pressed. It's uncertain why little attention has been given to this theory, but we have much to learn about Zika, and all avenues must be researched.

Unless we consider every alternative, we may be less effective in our ability to control the spread of both the Aedes mosquito and the Zika virus. If we are to have success in producing treatment or prevention options for this viral illness (none exists at present), we will have to take into account the chance that *this* Zika virus is not the same as the original.

Other Theories

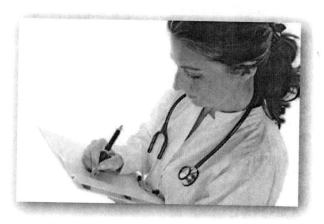

Whenever a new health risk is identified that might have epidemic consequences, the cause is often quickly identified. Almost as quickly as a reason for the outbreaks is found, however, a great number of alternative hypotheses begin circulating. Some of these may have basis in fact, but many are meant to play to the fear of the general population and, especially, conspiracy theorists.

There are a number of theories about the recent high numbers of microcephalic newborns that are reported in Zika epidemic zones. Some of these hypotheses have nothing to do with ZIKV at all. Everything from vaccines to the Rockefeller Foundation to Microsoft founder Bill Gates have been implicated.

The theories spring from reports in the Washington Post that not all babies in Brazil with microcephaly have been shown to be infected with Zika virus, and that some babies may have been born simply with abnormally small heads.

Experts scrutinized 732 cases they found that more than half either weren't microcephaly, or weren't related to Zika. Just 270 were confirmed as microcephaly that appears to be linked to Zika or other infectious diseases, according to a Brazilian health ministry bulletin.

Some scientists suggest that the new data means that Brazil will have fewer cases of Zika-related microcephaly than originally feared. Despite this claim, they have no alternative cause for why so many babies are born with abnormally small heads in the country. Over 4000 cases have been reported recently, while Brazil normally sees less than 150 in a year.

However, many other countries in the same region aren't reporting a large number of microcephalic newborns. Is it possible that Zika is not involved at all and is just coincidental to the recent explosion of birth defects in Brazil? It may, indeed, be the case.

The blogosphere is putting forth a number of alternative theories that "prove" that Zika virus is just a smokescreen for the real cause. Some make more sense than others.

One possible culprit, apparently, is Bill Gates. The Bill and Melinda Gates Foundation is involved in mosquito-borne disease control programs. The theory is that the Microsoft founder is associated with genetically-modified mosquitoes that have been released in Brazil and other countries that have had outbreaks of Dengue Fever, Malaria, Zika, and other illnesses.

THE GMO MOSQUITO THEORY:

The OX513A Aedes mosquito, mentioned earlier in this book, is an example of efforts to eliminate mosquito populations by inserting a GMO male mosquito that, when it mates with females, produces offspring that do not survive to adulthood. Other programs insert a large number of sterile males into the habitat which produce no offspring at all.

The OX513A mosquito, not actually related to Bill Gates but to a British company named Oxitec, has a gene that requires the antibiotic tetracycline to allow its offspring to survive. Theorists claim that a great deal of tetracycline is given to animals and can switch on the normal reproductive cycle in OX513A.

Perhaps, but the Aedes mosquito prefers human hosts, and there are no limit to them in a large, populous country like Brazil. In addition, the GMO mosquito released was not infected with Zika in the lab. In addition, as a male, OX513A does not bite humans at all.

Another fact is that the epicenter of the outbreak in Brazil is hundreds of miles from where the GMO male mosquitoes were released. Remember, these mosquitoes rarely travel more than a few hundred yards from where they were "born" during their entire lifetime.

In this case, it's hard to see a relation at all to the microcephaly cases except in the most convoluted manner possible: The mosquito is exposed to tetracycline from livestock in some way, and then passes DNA to a Zika-carrying female mosquito while mating. Mating somehow changes the virus's DNA and causes birth defects. This is pretty difficult to do, as Zika virus has no DNA; it's an RNA virus.

For those who are against GMO foods, it should be understood that the GMO OX513A male mosquito's effect on the environment is unlikely to be harmful. Remember that the Aedes mosquito is not a natural inhabitant of the New World. It is not meant to be there, and it may even be crowding out mosquito species that are natural denizens of the area.

Some conspiracy theories are harmless, but this one isn't. Oxitec's GM mosquito releases could potentially provide protection for millions of Brazilians not just from Zika but from other related mosquito-borne diseases like dengue and yellow fever as well. It could even protect visitors to the upcoming Summer Olympics in Rio de Janeiro.

Despite this, Brazilian authorities are already slowing down the release of the GMO mosquitoes due to public concern. When this happened in Nigeria some years ago, it seriously obstructed efforts to eradicate the dangerous viral disease Polio.

A LARVICIDE IS THE CAUSE

An Argentine physician's group called "Physicians in Crop-Sprayed Towns" believes that Zika is not involved at all in the surge of microcephalic infants in Brazil. They believe a Japanese-made larvicide named Pyriproxyfen is at fault.

The group points out that the grand majority of cases occur in one country, with nearby countries much less likely to see microcephaly despite plenty of acute Zika cases. Long-term exposure to Pyriproxyfen might cause effects on pregnancies that could lead to birth defects.

While it's true that ZIKV is seen in only a number of cases of microcephaly, the virus remains in the blood for only a week or so. It can be argued that the virus enters the body, does its damage, and disappears before tests can be performed.

Certainly, more study is needed before Zika can be proven as the cause of the abnormalities occurring in Brazil. However, we should see records of where and when this larvicide was used to show some likelihood for a possible link.

THE VACCINE-CAUSED PANDEMIC THEORY

Another theory blames a program encouraging pregnant women to get the vaccine against tetanus, diphtheria, and pertussis (Tdap vaccine). Instead of preventing medical problems, some say that the vaccine actually led to the increase in microcephaly in Brazilian babies. It's true that Guillain-Barre syndrome, also noted in the current epidemic in South America, may be a rare complication of certain vaccines. To some, this points to a vaccine as the cause.

Bill and Melinda Gates' foundation seems to have found its way into this theory too. It recently launched a study on the immune response of pregnant women to Tdap vaccine. Diabolical motives have been ascribed to the vaccine and some "ingredient" in it that causes microcephaly. Their feeling is that, in the Gates' attempt to decrease the surplus population of poor countries, the vaccine is the "cure" that will preserve world resources for the elite.

About Tdap vaccine and microcephaly: It's true that the vaccine is recommended during pregnancy, but it is normally given during the 27th to 36th week, well beyond the point that microcephaly would begin to occur. Most non-genetic causes of microcephaly other than Zika, such as German measles (Rubella), syphilis, or cytomegalovirus infections, affect pregnancies only if they are transmitted before 20 weeks.

Proponents of this theory point to a study by the Institute for Pure and Applied Knowledge (IPAK) in Allison Park, Pennsylvania. In the study, various theories favoring Tdap vaccine as the cause are put forth. It points to the fact that not all microcephalic newborns have evidence of the Zika virus. It points to, as we suggest in this book, a change in the genetics at one point where building blocks, known as amino acids, make the South American strain separate from those in the Old World.

It also points to the recent (2014) change in policy in some countries which recommends that pregnant women are candidates for the Tdap vaccine. A locally produced vaccine, "Boostrix", is cited as one version now put forth as mandatory in certain regions. Yet, IPAK states that no safety studies had been conducted on Tdap prior to the initiation of the Brazilian vaccination program.

One of their theories is that molecules in the "p" part of Tdap (pertussis, also known as "whooping cough") are, possibly, to blame. The researchers state that these molecules are similar to one or more human antigens involved in brain development. One is Toll-like receptor adaptor molecule 1 (TICAM1), which affects a protein involved in native immunity against invading pathogens.

Is there a reason to believe that the pertussis organism in Brazil is different from the one in the United States? A local mutation here might affect brain development even in later stages of the pregnancy.

To test a vaccine-related hypothesis, major studies looking at vaccinated versus unvaccinated pregnancies are warranted. Do unvaccinated women deliver babies that have microcephaly?

One issue with this theory is that the vaccine is routinely given in pregnancies throughout the world, including the United States. Yet, no increased numbers of microcephalic newborns have appeared there as they have in Brazil. In one study of over 36,000 pregnancies, Tdap vaccine given in a range of 1-40 weeks was not found to be associated with poor fetal outcomes.

VACCINE LOTS HAVE BEEN CONTAMINATED

The IPAK study also posited other theories as to why Zika may or may not be involved in the events in Brazil. One is the possible contamination of certain lots of vaccine with Pestivirus, a type of Bovine Viral Diarrhea virus. Reports of such contamination in vaccines used in livestock do exist, and one unrelated study in 2013 reported an increase in microcephaly (presumably in cattle).

As well, IPAK suggests that a compound known as Glyphosate in contaminated bovine products used in diet, vaccines, or elsewhere might have an effect. The researchers postulate that glyphosate may affect a protein (DNA-PKcs) involved in brain development. Defects as small as a single mutation in DNA-PKcs, they claim, may induce nervous system defects, including microcephaly.

In the United States, we are accustomed to stringent measures used to ensure purity of vaccines. Can the same be said of other countries? We certainly hope so, but the resources to assure purity of vaccines may not be available.

Human error was a clear factor in the spread of Ebola virus to two nurses in Texas; why couldn't human error play a part in contaminating an otherwise-benign vaccine? Further, why couldn't a contaminated vaccine have ill effects on those vaccinated or exposed in the womb?

Similarly, other products ingested during a pregnancy might affect the fetus. Excessive consumption of alcohol is well-known to cause Fetal Alcohol Syndrome, which can cause a number of defects. It's not unreasonable to evaluate the quality control in the production of vaccines and other products in countries affected by unusually high rates of microcephaly.

THE ZIKA VIRUS HAS SIMILAR GENETICS TO OTHER PROVEN VIRAL CAUSES OF MICROCEPHALY

In the last theory we'll explore that comes from the Institute of Pure and Applied Knowledge study, a relationship is suggested between the genome of the Zika virus and two viruses that have been proven to cause microcephaly if infected during times of significant brain growth and development in the womb.

Rubella (German measles) and cytomegalovirus are known to be associated with a higher rate of microcephaly. The IPAK study reviewed the makeup of these two viruses and compared it to that of ZIKV. They report a 47% congruency among the viruses' genetics, and suggest that this may relate to the possible tendency of Zika to cause effects on brain development.

THE ROCKEFELLER FOUNDATION SELLS THE VIRUS TO MAD SCIENTISTS

Another theory suggests that the Rockefeller Foundation, which may have acquired an interest, if not a patent, in the virus in the early 1950s, is responsible for releasing the virus into the environment. As a matter of fact, some say that the foundation didn't discover the virus in monkeys, but created it in a lab for later use.

It's true that the related American Type Culture Collection (ATCC) has a significant inventory of various micro-organisms. Although the foundation does, indeed, have samples of the virus for sale, their purpose is not domination of the planet, but to help aid research into the organism.

Let's say you wanted a sample of Zika virus for your own "use'. It's not as easy as ordering shirts online; you have to show major credentials and legal documents to indicate why it's important for you to obtain the virus. Having said that, if you were the chairman

of a university Infectious Disease Department, you could probably obtain a sample.

Unfortunately for this theory, a mad scientist or master criminal (with appropriate academic credentials and legal documents, of course) bent on world destruction would probably pick a virus that is historically more dangerous than ZIKV to release into society. How about Ebola, or just purchase a good supply of Anthrax? For those who believe Zika virus is a device for the control of the human population: If someone wanted to decimate the number of people on Earth, they could probably choose more dangerous viruses than ZIKV.

ZIKA VIRUS WAS RELEASED TO MAKE MONEY

Some even claim a financial motive for the current ZIKV pandemic. If a pharmaceutical company, Bill Gates, or the Rockefeller Foundation could spread the disease, a new vaccine could be developed that everyone throughout the world would have to buy. Drugs to treat the disease would be patented and sole control would go to the manufacturer.

To make a fortune from a non-existent vaccine (that probably won't be available for up to two years) might be a motivation for evil drug pushers like the pharmaceutical industry, but why cause a major health emergency before your drug or vaccine is ready for sale? There, apparently, needs to be more coordination between the research and sales departments. If this is what is happening, a CEO somewhere should be fired.

COMMON SENSE

Conspiracy theories will always circulate whenever a new health threat appears on the horizon. People who believe in them have an urgent sense that someone is out to get them; this sometimes borders on paranoia. Some of the scenarios envisioned could only come out of a science fiction movie.

Having said that, an open mind is essential. ZIKV could possibly be coincidental to the effects we're seeing on pregnancies, or there might be multiple factors involved. It seems easy to blame it all on the virus given the time frame, but sometimes there is much more below the surface.

Calm and rational thought, in combination with hard scientific data, should guide those who are searching for alternative causes for what is happening in Brazil and elsewhere. Pandemic disease is a serious problem, and we must be serious when we look for causes and treatments.

Our Policy Going Forward

The United States, so far, has been spared the heartbreaking consequences of widespread Zika outbreaks. The CDC has made statements about readiness policy in the face of ZIKV, something that was slowly instituted during the 2014 Ebola epidemic. Luckily, Ebola just barely touched our shores. The CDC has learned from the experience and wants to be sure the nation is prepared this time.

A prepared U.S. is good policy, but we must think beyond just fighting a possible Zika epidemic within our borders. The significant effect on the health and economies of many South American countries, mostly friendly to us, means that we must do more.

The economies of many of these nations are fragile, with many of them dependent upon our travel dollars. The CDC has issued warnings against pregnant women entering these countries, and that is wise advice. However, there must be a concerted effort to aid those expending scarce resources to keep their people (and their next generation) healthy.

This can be accomplished by helping augment mosquito control programs in the epidemic zone. We've got the funds and protocols to assist those desperately trying to contain Zika virus disease and its possible effect on newborns.

International cooperation is rarely discussed, but a thoughtful and articulate defense for helping those at risk comes from Mel Martinez, former senator of Florida, our most sub-tropical state; one that will surely be affected if Zika moves Northward in earnest. He said:

"The relationship between the United States and its closest neighbors is focused on economic and security matters. Concerns regarding health care rise to the top of the agenda only in times of crisis, and in those crises there are dangers as well as opportunities. So it is with the rapid proliferation of the Zika virus throughout the hemisphere.

In helping to lead a region-wide response, U.S. policymakers can improve the capacity of our neighbors to respond to this and future outbreaks, and in so doing better protect the American public and improve U.S. relations with Latin America."

Ex-senator Martinez also understands, as mentioned earlier in this book, the plight of less-developed countries. He wrote: "…In many countries, the poorest populations… have endured the brunt of this outbreak. These groups have traditionally not benefitted from economic development and investment in more affluent areas, and they are especially vulnerable now because of the scarcity of adequate health care in the areas where they live.

The Zika virus struck at a time when many nations in Latin America were looking towards new opportunities for economic growth and increased political stability. Cooperation will be key to mitigating the impact of this outbreak, and the effort to coordinate such a response can lay a foundation that will make all of the nations involved stronger, not weaker…"

We have a responsibility, as an exceptionally blessed nation, to help those under attack by Zika virus, and our leaders must work to alleviate the suffering of those less fortunate. By doing this, we'll decrease the chances of a major outbreak on our shores as well as ending the threat on theirs.

Now you know: Now you know how to best prevent the Zika virus from affecting you or your family. You learned the three D's of protection against mosquitoes and the illnesses they cause: Drain, Dress, and Defend. You know the various methods to eliminate both larvae and adults from your environment using source reduction, pesticides, and other weapons in your battle against mosquito-borne disease.

You also learned the best way to prevent Zika virus from affecting pregnant women and their fetuses, and what tests should be performed during pregnancy.

You additionally found out about some alternative theories about why (and if) ZIKV may be causing birth defects. Some have basis in fact and some don't. The controversies demonstrate why so much more research is still to be done before we are prepared to calmly deal with the possible effects of Zika virus or whatever other factor may be at work.

LAST THOUGHTS:

Like pandemics before it, the Zika virus must be approached without panic. The frightening nature of the birth defects and other possible complications of the disease require our attention, and our funding, to speed development of a vaccine and to prepare communities in the United States for possible outbreaks. We must exert our strongest efforts to prevent the heartbreak that comes when a family delivers a mentally-challenged newborn.

The World Health Organization is coordinating the efforts of many countries to combat ZIKV. With international cooperation, the world will best be able to control pandemic diseases. The U.S. has a history of success in these endeavors, once it understands the risks.

With the cooperation of the world's nations and their citizens, we can look forward to the day that Zika and other pandemic diseases may become just a bump in the road, and not the *end* of the road for humanity.

More information about Zika virus:
The Center for Disease Control and Prevention:
http://www.cdc.gov/zika/

The World Health Organization:
http://www.who.int/topics/zika/en/

Dr. Alton's medical preparedness website:
http://www.doomandbloom.net

CPSIA information can be obtained at www.ICGtesting.com
Printed in the USA
LVOW10s1800240516

489756LV00009B/251/P